Recent Advances in

Histopathology 24

Recent Advances in

Histopathology 24

Adrienne M Flanagan MD PhD FRCPath FMedSci
Professor of Musculoskeletal Pathology
Department of Pathology
University College London Cancer Institute, London, UK
Consultant Histopathologist
Department of Cellular and Molecular Pathology
Royal National Orthopaedic Hospital, Stanmore, UK

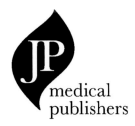

JP
medical
publishers

London • Philadelphia • Panama City • New Delhi

© 2016 JP Medical Ltd.
Published by JP Medical Ltd,
83 Victoria Street, London, SW1H 0HW, UK
Tel: +44 (0)20 3170 8910
Fax: +44 (0)20 3008 6180
Email: info@jpmedpub.com
Web: www.jpmedpub.com

ISBN: 978-1-909836-28-0

British Library Cataloguing in Publication Data
A catalogue record for this book is available from the British Library

Library of Congress Cataloging in Publication Data
A catalog record for this book is available from the Library of Congress

Commissioning Editor:	Steffan Clements
Editorial Assistant:	Adam Rajah
Design:	Designers Collective Ltd

Preface

It is with pleasure that I introduce volume 24 of *Recent Advances in Histopathology*.

The publication of the human genome sequence in 2001, and the technological advances that made it feasible and that have developed as a consequence of this milestone, have already impacted many areas of diagnostic histopathology, none more so than in cancer. The pathologist is no longer solely reliant on microscopic features for the classification of a disease, and can now provide more robust diagnoses by complementing a histological phenotype with molecular profiles. The spectrum of morphological features that have long been appreciated by pathologists can now be explained through DNA sequencing, opening up new avenues of research.

A number of chapters in this book capture the transformational changes that are occurring in our discipline, and will therefore be of interest to the pathologist, the generalist, the specialist who wishes to remain abreast of recent changes in the field, and those preparing for their postgraduate exams. There are also two chapters covering postmortem pathology, which demonstrate how the study of the cause of death remains a much needed and valuable resource.

If the technological advances in biomedical science that have taken place over the last two decades are to be exploited effectively, change is required in medical education. It was with this in mind that Professor Davinder Sandhu was commissioned to provide a comprehensive overview of postgraduate education in the UK.

I wish to thank all of the contributors who kindly gave up their time, and I am grateful to Steffan Clements, the commissioning editor, for his support throughout the project.

Adrienne Flanagan
August 2016

Contents

Chapter 1

Pathology of acute lung injury

William AH Wallace

INTRODUCTION

The term acute lung injury (ALI) means different things to different specialist groups. In respiratory medicine and intensive care, ALI is part of a clinical spectrum of lung injury up to and including the adult respiratory distress syndrome (ARDS). This was defined in 1994 by a joint American and European Consensus Conference [1] as a condition with acute onset, bilateral pulmonary infiltrates on chest X-ray/CT, impaired oxygenation and the absence of left atrial hypertension. Oxygenation was assessed as the ratio between Pao_2 (the partial pressure of oxygen in arterial blood) and Fio_2 (the fraction of oxygen in the inspired air), and in a clinical setting a ratio of <300 mmHg was consistent with a diagnosis of ARDS, while less severe injury with a ratio of <200 mmHg was termed ALI. In 2012, a revision of this was published by the ARDS Definition Task Force [2]. This defined ARDS as having onset within 1 week of a clinical insult, bilateral radiological opacities and an objective demonstration that lung oedema was not hydrostatic in nature. They divided cases into mild, moderate or severe ARDS on the basis of the Pao_2/Fio_2 ratio with the term ALI no longer being used.

In the pathology literature, the term 'acute lung injury' was also put forward by Katzenstein to describe inflammatory/fibroblastic processes in lungs that are felt to be of acute onset with temporal homogeneity, usually characterised by loose oedematous 'granulation tissue' like stroma reflecting response to an insult occurring at one point in time [3]. The aim was to differentiate these conditions from the chronic interstitial pneumonias that had a longer time course and showed mature fibrosis. This pathological definition is broader than the clinical definition and includes a range of patterns of lung remodelling including diffuse alveolar damage syndrome (DADS) as seen in patients with ALI/ARDS, as well as some other patterns of lung injury such as cryptogenic organising pneumonia (COP) and eosinophilic pneumonia. In addition, the recent American Thoracic Society/European Respiratory Society consensus statement on the classification of idiopathic interstitial pneumonias has suggested that the clinical term 'acute interstitial pneumonitis' (AIP) should be adopted in cases of idiopathic lung injury with a DADS pattern on histology [4] adding yet another layer to the terminology.

This chapter will focus on the pathology of the clinical syndrome of ALI/ARDS looking at the aetiology, the pathological features and the pathogenesis, as currently understood. The potential issues to be considered, difficulties and differential diagnoses that may be

William AH Wallace BSc (Hons) MBChB (Hons) PhD FRCPEd FRCPath, Consultant Pathologist, Department of Pathology, Royal Infirmary of Edinburgh, UK. Email: william.wallace@luht.scot.nhs.uk (for correspondence)

encountered when these patients undergo lung biopsy for histological evaluation or come to autopsy will then be discussed.

AETIOLOGY

ALI/ARDS may be idiopathic (AIP) or arise in the context of a wide range of primary pulmonary conditions as well as representing a complication of numerous extra-pulmonary insults [5] (**Table 1.1**). Although subtle differences exist between cases associated with pulmonary and non-pulmonary causes [6], the pathological features, at least at the level we currently understand them, are sufficiently uniform that this can be regarded as a stereotypical pattern of lung injury. What is very clear, however, is the importance of both pulmonary and systemic sepsis as a trigger. Clinical studies have indicated that this is the pre-eminent risk factor and prompt and early recognition of this is essential in reducing the incidence of ALI/ARDS [7].

It is, however, important to acknowledge that the development of ALI/ARDS is not inevitable, even in patients with recognised risk factors, suggesting that there are 'host factors' that predispose some patients to develop the syndrome. This has led to searches for genetic factors and biomarkers that predict both susceptibility and severity of lung injury [8,9]. It is also becoming increasing recognised that DADS can present as an acute exacerbation with respiratory failure on a background of idiopathic pulmonary fibrosis/usual interstitial pneumonitis (IPF/UIP) [10].

THE HISTOLOGICAL FEATURES OF ALI/ARDS

The pathological pattern of lung abnormality encountered in patients with ALI/ARDS is termed DADS [11–13]. Traditionally, this is divided into three phases, but it is important

Table 1.1 Causes of ALI/ARDS		
Direct lung injury	**Indirect lung injury**	**Idiopathic**
Pneumonia (bacterial, viral, fungal) Inhalation injury, e.g. gastric contents, smoke, corrosive vapours such as ammonia Therapeutic drug reactions, e.g. bleomycin and methotrexate Pulmonary contusion/blast injury Fat emboli Near-drowning Reperfusion/re-expansion lung injury (including postlung transplant) Radiation injury Altitude (acute mountain sickness)	Systemic sepsis especially with gram-negative bacilli Major extra thoracic trauma with or without fat emboli Acute pancreatitis Drug overdose, e.g. opiates and barbiturates Transfusion of blood products Disseminated intravascular coagulation Systemic poisoning, e.g. paraquat Eclampsia	Acute interstitial pneumonitis
ALI/ARDS can be associated with a wide range of pulmonary and non-pulmonary conditions. It is important, however, to realise that it may be a rare complication in many of these situations suggesting that other contributing factors, including host factors, may be important in the development of lung injury. In some instances, similar clinical features with pathological evidence of diffuse alveolar damage syndrome may be seen that appears idiopathic. In this instance, the clinical term 'acute interstitial pneumonitis' (AIP) is preferred. Reprinted with permission from Hasleton et al [11].		

to recognise that these represent a continuous process rather than distinct steps. The early events comprise an 'exudative' phase that is followed by a 'proliferative' phase. In some patients, this is followed by resolution of the fibroproliferative process with the lung architecture returning to normal or near normal but in many patients the process is progressive with the development of fibrosis. As would be expected each 'phase' is complex and our understanding in many ways remains limited but as will be discussed later, we are gaining some understanding of the cellular and inflammatory mediators involved.

Exudative phase

In the early stage of the exudative phase, the lungs appear macroscopically normal but as the process develops the lungs become oedematous. Autopsy examination of patients dying at this stage characteristically show lungs that are heavy (>1 kg) with a red, beefy appearance, and are firm on palpation (**Figure 1.1**). The earliest changes are not seen by light microscopy but electron microscopic studies demonstrate necrosis of type I alveolar epithelial cells with a denuded basement membrane, increased numbers of marginated neutrophils in the alveolar capillaries with, in some cases, fibrin thrombi and interstitial oedema.

Two to three days from the onset of injury, oedema becomes apparent at the light microscopic level. This exudative oedema fluid, often with associated haemorrhage, is rich in fibrin and fills the alveolar spaces becoming mixed with necrotic debris. The fibrin condenses to form the characteristic histological feature of the exudative phase – a hyaline membrane (**Figure 1.2**). Initially, these may be relatively localised but as the injury develops they become more widely seen. The hyaline membranes appear on haematoxylin and eosin staining as intensely eosinophilic bands of proteinaceous material lining the alveolar airspaces and ducts. Significant numbers of inflammatory cells within the interstitium or alveolar spaces are not a conspicuous feature although neutrophils are believed to have a critical role in the pathogenesis of ALI/ARDS. In cases where significant numbers of neutrophils are evident, particularly in the alveolar spaces associated with fibrinous exudates, the possibility of pneumonia needs to be considered recognising that both can coexist.

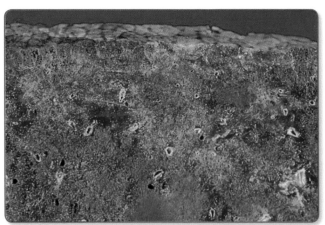

Figure 1.1 Macroscopic appearance of a fixed lung slice demonstrating the appearance of the lung in the exudative phase of diffuse alveolar damage syndrome. The cut surface of the lung is red, congested and firm. The process is generally diffuse but in some cases can be more localised. By courtesy of Prof DB Fleider, Philadelphia, USA. Reprinted with permission from Hasleton et al [11].

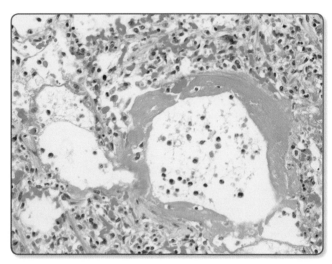

Figure 1.2 Histologically the exudative phase is characterised by the presence of hyaline membranes. These are dense eosinophillic bands that line the alveolar space and represent condensed proteinaceous fluid. Small numbers of neutrophils and other inflammatory cells may be seen but if large numbers are present the possibility of pneumonia should be considered. Reprinted with permission from Hasleton et al [11].

Proliferative phase

Histological features in keeping with the development of the proliferative phase are usually seen 5–7 days from the onset of lung injury. Macroscopically the lungs remain heavy but show a grey, consolidated firm appearance (**Figure 1.3**). The characteristic feature of the proliferative phase is the progression to organisation of the exudate. Ultrastructural studies have demonstrated that the basement membrane is further disrupted. Myofibroblasts proliferate both within the interstitium and also migrate through the breaks in the basement membrane into the exudates, giving rise to the development of granulation tissue within alveolar spaces and ducts (**Figure 1.4**). In the early stages, this may be patchy in its distribution and coexist with persisting hyaline membranes in keeping with the concept that this is an evolving process. The organisation of the luminal exudates is accompanied by prominent proliferation of type II alveolar cells along the alveolar walls. These have a cuboidal, 'hob-nail' appearance and may show significant cytological atypia with pleomorphic nuclei and large punctuate nucleoli.

Fibrotic phase

In most cases, the proliferative stage is followed by organisation with progressive interstitial fibrosis, collapse of the alveolar architecture and distortion of the lung architecture. Examination of the lungs at autopsy from patients with DADS who survive several weeks following onset of ALI/ARDS can show various patterns of established fibrosis. In some cases, the lungs may show extensive sheets of fibrosis, occasionally with honeycombing. Other areas of fibrosis may be more nodular with entrapped cleft-like spaces lined by alveolar epithelial cells, while in some instances a more diffuse, less destructive pattern of alveolar wall thickening that resembles fibrotic nonspecific interstitial pneumonitis may be apparent. It is important to realise that different patterns may be observed in sections taken from different areas of the same lung. In cases with prominent honeycomb or subpleural fibrosis, the possibility that this represents DADS superimposed on a background of IPF needs to be considered (see below). In addition to the fibrosis, there is often evidence of extensive squamous metaplasia, secondary inflammatory changes and evidence of

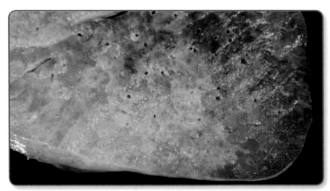

Figure 1.3 Macroscopic appearance of a fixed lung slice demonstrating the appearance of the lung in the proliferative phase of diffuse alveolar damage syndrome. The lung shows rather irregular foci of grey, firm 'consolidation.' By courtesy of Prof Fleider DB, Philadelphia, USA. Reprinted with permission from Hasleton et al [11].

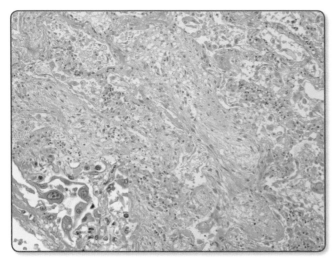

Figure 1.4 Histologically the proliferative phase is characterised by the development of extensive buds of organising fibroblastic tissue in the alveolar spaces. This may be admixed with identifiable hyaline membranes in keeping with diffuse alveolar damage syndrome being a dynamic process rather than a series of discreet events. Insert demonstrates the presence of marked epithelial atypia that may raise concerns about the possibility of malignancy, especially in cytology specimens. Reprinted with permission from Hasleton et al [11].

vascular remodelling with extensive hypertrophy of the media and irregular intimal fibrosis.

While the majority of patients with ALI/ARDS who survive long enough show evidence of fibrosis, there are a group of patients in which the proliferative phase undergoes resolution, either in part or in some cases, totally. These patients may be left with minimal respiratory symptoms although some impairment in lung function can be seen, particularly in carbon monoxide diffusing capacity, suggesting that even in these patients some degree of alveolar fibrosis has occurred.

PATHOGENESIS OF ALI/ARDS

Traditionally the pathogenetic processes that are associated with the development of ALI/ARDS are divided into the same phases as the histological changes. This, however, represents an over simplification, and there is evidence that fibroproliferation and attempts at healing occur simultaneously with the injurious processes that characterise the early exudative phase [14]. The following represents an overview of the pathogenesis and further more detailed information is available in reviews of the subject [11,15–19].

Exudative phase

A sustained inflammatory insult principally mediated by neutrophils and characterised by pulmonary capillary endothelial and alveolar epithelial cell injury is believed to be the hallmark of ALI. There is evidence to indicate neutrophil trapping in the pulmonary circulation at an early stage in the disease process and increased numbers can be recovered in bronchoalveolar lavage fluid supporting a central role for these cells in the injury phase. It is, however, important to note that ALI can also occur in neutropaenic patients.

IL-8, other members of the chemokine family, pro-inflammatory mediators such as C5a and leukotrienes, as well as bacterial endotoxin, have all been identified as being important in the recruitment, activation and retention of neutrophils in the pulmonary circulation. The mechanism whereby this occurs is thought to be by a combination of passive and active events. There is decreased neutrophil deformability resulting in an impaired ability of these cells to pass through the capillary bed of the lung. In addition, neutrophils are actively retained following activation of the pulmonary endothelial cells, an event that occurs early in the process. This is driven by IL-1 and TNFα and results in increased expression of endothelial adhesion molecules such as selectins and intercellular adhesion molecule 1 allowing neutrophil attachment and margination via β2 integrins expressed on their cell surface.

Simultaneously chemokines, such as IL-8 and other pro-inflammatory cytokines, including IL-1, IL-6 and macrophage migration inhibitory factor (MIF), are released further promoting recruitment and retention of inflammatory cells. In addition, neutrophil turnover and survival in the lung also appears to be dysregulated. The normal mechanism whereby neutrophils recruited by inflammatory signals undergo apoptosis appears disrupted, and it is believed that neutrophils recruited to the lung in ALI are more resistant to apoptosis, thereby potentiating the tissue damage.

Resident tissue macrophages in the lung tissue can be activated by exposure to bacterial products such as lipopolysaccharide (LPS) and by cytokines such as MIF. These cells are important sources of primary inflammatory cytokines such as IL-1 TNFα, IL-8 and MIF that means they may have a role in amplifying the inflammatory processes as well as contributing directly to tissue damage that may in part explain why ALI can occur in neutropenic patients. The activation of neutrophils and resident macrophages results in release of a wide range of biologically active molecules including proteolytic enzymes (neutrophil elastase, collagenases and gelatinases), reactive oxygen species, leukotrienes and platelet activating factor that damage the overlying alveolar epithelial cells and the basement membrane.

Endothelial cell injury is mediated by a wide range of potential triggers. Among the most important are cytokines, especially TNFα and IL-1, vascular endothelial growth factor (VEGF), bacterial products, such as LPS, immune complexes, radiation and ischaemia/reperfusion. This promotes changes in cell morphology as well as potentiating a proinflammatory, prothrombotic environment with increased production of thromboxane A_2, platelet activating factor and endothelin-1 as well as a reduction in prostaglandin I_2.

The change in endothelial cell morphology is brought about by cellular contraction and results in a permissive fluid shift between the circulation and the extravascular space via gaps which develop between the endothelial cells, through which fluid and macromolecules can escape. This increase in lung vascular permeability results in the movement of fluid with a high protein content into the alveolar interstitium. Type I pneumocytes on the other side of the alveolar basement membrane form a tight barrier, which in health prevents the passive movement of fluid from the interstitium into the alveolar space. In addition to this passive role in maintaining the integrity of the alveolar space, these cells also play an active role in preventing fluid accumulation in the lung via Na^+/K^+ ion transport channels and aquaporins. The latter are believed to allow movement of water across these cells in a manner independent of ionic pumping. In ALI, there is damage to this alveolar epithelial barrier with cellular necrosis and denudation of the basement membrane such that this barrier is lost.

From the discussion above, a sequence of events can be postulated to explain the exudative phase. Neutrophil activation and retention in the lung occurs in tandem with endothelial injury/activation promoting a proinflammatory environment as well as allowing fluid and inflammatory cells to move into the interstitium. Associated epithelial injury allows this fluid into the alveolar spaces. This increase in fluid within the alveoli may initially be counteracted by an increase in fluid transport out of the alveoli via the Na^+/K^+ pumps and the aquaporins, but this requires functional epithelium. As the degree of epithelial injury increases, this capacity is degraded and the alveoli become flooded with the protein-rich oedema fluid.

Fibroproliferative phase

As has been discussed above this phase is characterised by the migration of myofibroblasts into the exudate fluid in alveolar spaces, with subsequent proliferation, deposition of extracellular matrix proteins and angiogenesis, giving rise to loose granulation tissue formation. This is associated with prominent type II pneumocyte proliferation. These are believed to represent the alveolar epithelial stem cell population and this represents evidence for an attempt at alveolar healing.

Although this process is usually regarded as following on from the exudative phase, it may in fact start early in the process as BAL fluid obtained from patients even in the earliest stages of ALI shows increased mitogenic activity for fibroblasts in vitro. This process is believed to be mediated principally by macrophage-derived factors such as platelet-derived growth factor, insulin-like growth factor-1, basic fibroblast growth factor and TGFβ1. The recruitment of myofibroblasts into the alveolar space is associated with secretion of extracellular matrix proteins including fibronectin, tenascin and collagen III. This is associated with accumulation of mucopolysaccharides, such as hyaluronic acid, giving rise to the loose myxoid appearance that characterises the plugs of material forming in the alveolar sacs. Regulation of the angiogenesis that accompanies this process is less well understood. Possible roles for IL-8, monocyte-derived CXC chemokines, VEGF and procollagens have all been suggested.

Regulation of the epithelial proliferation appears to involve signalling between epithelial cells in autocrine and paracrine fashions as well as through direct interaction between these cells and elements in the extracellular matrix. BAL fluid from patients even in the early phase of ALI promotes epithelial proliferation in vivo. A variety of epithelial mitogens including by IL-1β, TGFα, keratinocyte growth factor and hepatocyte growth factor have been implicated as having a possible role in this. One important function of re-epithelialisation is that the presence of epithelial cells on the basement membrane appears to inhibit fibroblast proliferation, although the mechanism of this is unclear.

Fibrosis versus resolution

The regulation of wound healing in other tissues has been extensively studied. In dermal wounds, the granulation tissue undergoes organisation with the development of increasingly mature fibrous tissue that remodels eventually forming a scar predominantly composed of collagen I. In many patients with ALI/ARDS, an analogous process occurs with deposition of collagen resulting in the lungs becoming scarred with impaired function. In some cases, the pre-existing architecture may still be recognisable but the individual alveolar walls are diffusely thickened giving rise to a nonspecific interstitial pneumonia like pattern. In other cases, the lung architecture appears to collapse entirely and is replaced by sheets of fibrous tissue.

The process described above could be regarded as the expected outcome, given the normal progression of granulation tissue to scar formation that occurs at sites of tissue injury but intriguingly in some patients with ALI the fibro-proliferative component may either, in part, or more rarely wholly resolve. In these instances the lung architecture returns to a normal or near normal appearance. The regulation of this process is very poorly understood, but it must involve cessation of the process that initiated ALI, removal of oedema fluid and fibroproliferative granulation tissue from the alveolar spaces as well as re-epithelialisation of the alveoli and repair of endothelial damage.

Cessation of the inflammatory process by removal of the triggering event is likely to reduce neutrophil and macrophage activation as well as decreasing endothelial and epithelial injury. This may be associated with increased neutrophil apoptosis in the lung. In addition, many of the pro-inflammatory agents discussed above have natural tissue inhibitors and the environment in the tissues may shift from being pro-injury and fibrosis to pro-resolution. Oedema fluid may be cleared by the proliferating alveolar epithelial cells while the granulation tissue may be removed by a combination of myofibroblast apoptosis and metalloproteinase (MMP) digestion of the extracellular matrix. BAL fluid from patients with resolving ALI has been shown to initiate apoptosis in fibroblasts in vitro and MMP-2 and MMP-9 are increased in the lungs of patients with ALI. Epithelial proliferation has been discussed above and as this progresses the type II cells differentiate and flatten out to form new type I cells. Very little is known about repair of the capillaries, but it is assumed that there is endothelial proliferation and that fibrin thrombi are removed by the fibrinolytic system.

In this context, it is important to acknowledge that unlike the liver there is no evidence the lung can reconstitute itself following extensive tissue destruction. This means that for resolution to occur the elastic and collagen scaffolding of the lung remain must remain intact so that healing of individual alveolar spaces can occur. If severe tissue injury occurs and the alveolar structure is destroyed then fibrosis may be the inevitable outcome [20]. This concept would fit with clinical studies that have found that markers of inflammatory damage to the lung correlate with clinical outcome.

THE ROLE OF PATHOLOGICAL DIAGNOSIS IN ALI/ARDS

As has been discussed above, ALI/ARDS is essentially a clinical diagnosis and pathological assessment is not usually required. The most common specimens likely to be encountered from these patients are bronchoscopic lavage samples that have been taken to identify potential infective organisms in the lung and these are frequently also submitted for diagnostic cytology [21]. As has been discussed above, the regenerating alveolar epithelial cells present in the distal lung can show severe reactive cytological atypia and great care needs to be taken to avoid an erroneous diagnosis of malignancy.

Surgical lung biopsies are not frequently performed but may be done when there is clinical uncertainty around the diagnosis [22,23]. The histological features will clearly depend on the stage of the process at which the biopsy is taken. The principal differential diagnoses to consider histologically are those which may show some morphological overlap with DADS. These include organising pneumonia, eosinophillic pneumonia, acute hypersensitivity pneumonitis and occasionally vasculitis (polyangiitis with granulomatosis/ Wegener's granulomatosis when this is associated with a prominent organising pneumonic component and microscopic polyangiitis with extensive lung haemorrhage) [12]. In more chronic cases with established fibrosis variable patterns of remodelling may be seen and the possibility of fibrotic nonspecific interstitial pneumonitis or UIP may need to be considered. It is critical in these cases to have good clinical-radiological-pathological correlation with multidisciplinary discussion in order to establish a diagnosis especially as some of these may be amenable to specific therapeutic interventions with a better outlook than DADS.

More recently a further pattern of ALI, acute fibrinous organising pneumonia (AFOP) has been described [24]. This pattern may be idiopathic but can be seen in association with connective tissue disorders, infection, drug reactions and in patients with malignancy. Patients typically present with a short history of increasing breathlessness and cough and may have respiratory failure requiring ventilation. Histologically, the lung shows the presence of fibrinous balls within the alveolar spaces with variable evidence of organisation. Hyaline membranes are however not seen (**Figure 1.5**). The process is patchy in the lung and inflammatory cells are usually sparse. Some of these patients show a rapid progression to death, while others have a more subacute course and survive.

The commonest situation in which ALI/ARDS is encountered in routine diagnostic practice is, however, in the hospital autopsy [25,26]. The patient typically has been admitted to ITU in respiratory failure, where a clinical diagnosis has been made and the patient has then died some hours, days or even weeks later. Frustratingly in these cases the autopsy often adds very little other than confirming the presence of DADS with variable evidence of fibrosis. Tissue should be submitted for bacterial, fungal and viral cultures but these are often negative and the significance of any positive results may be unclear given that these patients are at risk of secondary ventilator associated pneumonias.

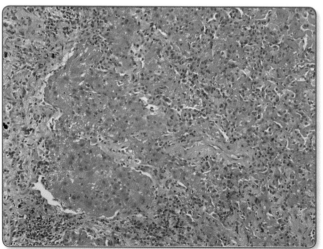

Figure 1.5 Acute fibrinous organising pneumonia is characterised by the accumulation of fibrin within alveolar spaces without hyaline membrane formation.

As has been discussed already DADS can be seen as an acute complication of IPF/UIP [4,10] (**Figure 1.6**). In many instances, there is a clinical history of this, but in some cases, this may be the first presentation with the underlying IPF/UIP having been unrecognised. It is important to examine such lungs carefully looking for any macroscopic and microscopic evidence of more established mature, honeycomb pattern of fibrosis with a subpleural and basal distribution. This usually involves taking multiple blocks from each lobe remembering to include the subpleural region. In some cases, underlying UIP may be relatively easy to differentiate from the more acute superimposed DADS but in others, particularly when the DADS is becoming more fibrotic this may be very difficult. Careful review of radiology at the time of first presentation may help as the finding of established fibrosis at that time would suggest an underlying more chronic condition.

SUMMARY

ALI/ARDS represents a complex clinical problem, and while there has been some improvement in survival, it still has a 40–50% mortality although this is showing some improvement [27,28]. Clinical management remains supportive; treating the underlying cause, often sepsis, and attempting to optimise oxygenation without inducing further ventilator associated injury to the lung. It does, however, represent an interesting 'model' of lung injury and remodelling in that the fibrotic process appears to be subject to factors that induce resolution rather than progression. While we have only a very superficial understanding of this currently, further elucidation of these mechanisms may provide therapeutic targets relevant to a broad range of progressive fibrotic lung diseases and not just ALI/ARDS.

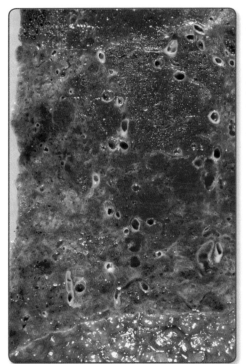

Figure 1.6 Macroscopic appearance of diffuse alveolar damage syndrome (DADS) that has developed on a background of known idiopathic pulmonary fibrosis. Most of the cut lung surface shows the typical red, beefy pattern typical of the exudative phase of DADS. In addition, however, there is evidence of pale subpleural fibrous tissue that represents the previous established fibrosis of usual interstitial pneumonitis. By courtesy of Prof KM Kerr, Aberdeen, UK. Reprinted with permission from Hasleton et al [11].

Key points for clinical practice

- ALI/ARDS is a clinically defined condition that represents a broadly stereotypical pattern of lung injury secondary to a wide range of pulmonary and extrapulmonary insults that is associated with around a 40–50% mortality.

- DADS represents the pathological pattern of injury most commonly seen in patients with ALI/ARDS.

- Although advances have been made in understanding the pathogenesis of ALI/ARDS, particularly the injury phase, much remains unclear especially in relation to the regulation of progressive fibrosis versus resolution. An improved understanding of how immature fibroblastic remodelling in the lung can be reversed may have importance in other progressive fibrotic lung conditions.

REFERENCES

1. Bernard GR, Artigas A, Brigham KL, et al. Report of the American-European consensus conference on ARDS: definitions, mechanisms, relevant outcomes and clinical trial coordination. Paris, Intensive Care Med 1994; 20:225–232.
2. The ARDS Definition Task Force. Acute Respiratory Distress Syndrome: the Berlin definition. Chicago, JAMA 2012; 307:2526–2533.
3. Katzenstein AL. Acute lung injury patterns: diffuse alveolar damage and bronchiolitis-obliterans-organising pneumonia. In: Katzenstin and Askin's Surgical pathology of nonneoplastic lung disease, 4th edn. Philadelphia, PA: WB Saunders, 2006:17–50.
4. Travis WD, Costabel U, Hansell DM, et al. on behalf of the ATS/ERS Committee on Idiopathic Interstitial Pneumonias. An official American Thoracic Society/European Respiratory Society statement: update of the international multidisciplinary classification of idiopathic interstitial pneumonias. New York: Am J Resp Crit Care Med 2013; 166:733–748.
5. Ware LB, Matthay MA. The acute respiratory distress syndrome. Massachusetts, N Engl J Med 2000; 342:1334–1349.
6. Rocco PR, Pelosi P. Pulmonary and extrapulmonary acute respiratory distress syndrome: myth or reality? London, Curr Opin Crit Care 2008; 14:50–55.
7. Dellinger RP, Levy MM, Carlet JM, et al. Surviving Sepsis Campaign: international guidelines for management of severe sepsis and septic shock: 2008. Crit Care Med 2008; 36:296–327.
8. Gao L, Barnes KC. Recent advances in genetic predisposition to clinical acute lung injury. Am J Physiol Lung Cell Mol Physiol 2009; 296:L713– L725.
9. Janz DR, Ware LB. Biomarkers of ALI/ARDS: pathogenesis, discovery and relevance to clinical trials. Semin Respir Crit Care Med 2013; 34:537–548.
10. Bouros D, Nicholson AC, Polychronopoulos V, et al. Acute interstitial pneumonia. Eur Respir J 2000; 15:412–418.
11. Wallace WAH, Simpson AJ, Hirani N. Acute lung injury. In: Hasleton P, Flieder DB (eds), Spencer's pathology of the lung, 6th edn. Cambridge: Cambridge University Press, 2013:342–365.
12. Beasley MB. Acute lung injury. In: Tomashefski JF, Cagle PT, Farver CF and Fraire AE (eds), Dail and Hammar's pulmonary pathology, Vol. 1, 3rd edn. New York: Springer, 2008:64–83.
13. Tomashefski JF. Pulmonary pathology of acute respiratory distress syndrome. Clin Chest Med 2000; 21:435–466.
14. Marshall RP, Bellingan G, Webb S, et al. Fibroproliferation occurs early in the acute respiratory distress syndrome and impacts on outcome. Am J Respir Crit Care Med 2000; 162:1783–1788.
15. Ware LB. Pathophysiology of acute lung injury and the adult respiratory distress syndrome. Semin Respir Crit Care Med 2006; 27:337–349.
16. Matthay MA, Zemans RL. The acute respiratory distress syndrome: pathogenesis and treatment. Annu Rev Pathol 2011; 6:147–163.
17. Schwarz MA. Acute lung injury: cellular mechanisms and derangements. Paediatr Respir Rev 2001; 2:3–9.

18. Pugin J, Verghese G, Widmer M-C, et al. The alveolar space is the site of intense inflammatory and profibrotic reactions in the early phase of ARDS. Am Rev Resp Dis 1997; 272:L442–L451.

19. Orfanos SE, Mavrommati I, Korovesi I, et al. Pulmonary endothelium in acute lung injury: from basic science to the critically ill. Intensive Care Med 2004; 30:1702–1714.

20. Wallace WAH, Fitch PM, Simpson AJ, et al. Inflammation associated remodelling and fibrosis in the lung – a process and an end point. Int J Exp Path 2007; 88:103–110.

21. Meduri GU, Chastre J. The standardisation of bronchoscopic techniques for ventilator-associated pneumonia. Chest 1992; 102:557S–564S.

22. Patel SR, Karmpaliotis D, Ayas NT, et al. The role of open-lung biopsy in ARDS. Chest 2004; 125:197–202.

23. Papazian L, Doddoli C, Chetaille B, et al. A contributive result of open-lung biopsy improves survival in acute respiratory distress syndrome patients. Crit Care Med 2007; 35:755–762.

24. Beasley MB, Franks TJ, Galvin JR, et al. Acute fibrinous and organising pneumonia: a histological pattern of lung injury and possible variant of diffuse alveolar damage. Arch Pathol Lab Med 2002; 126:1064–1070.

25. Ferguson ND, Frutos-Vivar F, Esteban A, et al. Acute respiratory distress syndrome: underrecognition by clinicians and diagnostic accuracy of three clinical definitions. Crit Care Med 2005; 33:2228–2234.

26. Esteban A, Fernández-Segoviano P, Frutos-Vivar F, et al. Comparison of clinical criteria for the acute respiratory distress syndrome with autopsy findings. Ann Intern Med 2004; 141:440–445.

27. Zambon M, Vincent JL. Mortality rates for patients with acute lung injury/ARDS have decreased over time. Chest 2008; 133:1120–1127.

28. MacCallum NS, Evans TW. Epidemiology of acute lung injury. Curr Opin Crit Care 2005; 11:43–49.

Chapter 2

Molecular profiling of breast cancer

Emad A Rakha, Ian O Ellis

INTRODUCTION

Traditionally, breast cancer has been classified by tumour stage. Morphological features, namely histological tumour type, tumour grade, proliferation status and lymphovascular invasion, have also been recognised as important prognostic variables [1,2].

We now know that breast cancer is caused by a heterogeneous group of tumours, and that tumour behaviour and response to therapy is determined by underlying biological features. The widespread use of mammographic screening, the greater availability of systemic therapy options and the move towards precision medicine drove the transition from purely prognostic classification systems to those predict the response to various therapeutic modalities. The current morphological surrogates based on the anatomical and histological properties of the tumour do not, however, reflect the biological and molecular heterogeneity of breast cancer, nor do they fully explain the genetic abnormalities found in tumours. Therefore, the importance of finding molecular biomarkers that predict behaviour and response to therapy is increasingly recognised.

Gene expression profiling

The first molecular classification systems employed a limited number of biomarkers, namely hormone receptors and HER2 which predicted the response to hormone therapy and anti-HER2-targeted therapy respectively. Although these markers showed prognostic significance, their clinical application was based on their predictive value. With the introduction of high-throughput molecular technology, it became possible to conduct simultaneous analyses of the expression of thousands of genes in a single experiment. Using unsupervised clustering techniques, breast cancer was grouped into clusters or intrinsic subtypes based on the quantitative expression of several genes (transcriptome profiles). These molecular subtypes were recognised to be associated with the outcome of therapy [3,4].

Emad A Rakha FRCPath, Department of Histopathology, Division of Cancer and Stem Cells, School of Medicine, University of Nottingham and Nottingham University Hospital NHS Trust, Nottingham City Hospital, Nottingham, UK.
Email: emadrakha@yahoo.com (for correspondence)

Ian O Ellis FRCPath, Department of Histopathology, Division of Cancer and Stem Cells, School of Medicine, University of Nottingham and Nottingham University Hospital NHS Trust, Nottingham City Hospital, Nottingham, UK.

Although genome-wide microarray-based gene expression profiling (GEP) studies provided further evidence to support the hypothesis that oestrogen receptor (ER) and HER2 are the key determinants of the molecular profiles of breast cancers, the studies also showed that these two biomarkers alone were unable to explain the heterogeneity of breast cancer. This technology in fact provided a molecular explanation for breast cancer heterogeneity observed at the clinicopathological level. For instance, the luminal ER-positive class, which comprises approximately 70% of breast cancers, shows a heterogeneous clinical outcome and a variable response to systemic therapy. It has been documented in ER-positive breast cancer that hormone therapy reduces a 10-year recurrence rate by approximately 50% and reduces a 15-year mortality by a third [5]; however, a proportion of ER-positive tumours did not respond [6], indicating that other genes and pathways are involved in determining the response and behaviour of these tumours.

Currently available variables have limited predictive value, emphasising the need to identify molecular assays and gene signatures that determine the outcome and response to therapy more precisely. Therefore, the introduction of GEP techniques has provided hope that the molecular profiling of breast cancer can be used to predict outcome and response to treatment. Subsequent studies demonstrated not only an association between molecular intrinsic subtype classification and outcome and response to therapy, but they have also indicated that different pathways are active in certain subtypes, making them potential candidates for targeted therapy.

Although GEP-based molecular subtyping shows promise, its application in routine practice has been less successful because of the cost, access to the technology and the need for fresh tumour material. Subsequently, replicating microarray-based molecular 'intrinsic subtype' classification systems have been developed. These use more available technology, including reverse transcription polymerase chain reaction (RT-PCR), and immunohistochemistry (IHC) which utilises a limited number of biomarkers. More recently, molecular intrinsic subtyping that uses formalin-fixed paraffin-embedded (FFPE) material has become available [7].

Despite the limited clinical use of molecular intrinsic subtyping and class discovery studies, GEP technology has opened new avenues for the molecular prognostication of breast cancer and the prediction of response to therapy. Importantly, it led to the introduction of molecular multigene assays that aim to classify subgroups of breast cancer based on the outcome or response to different therapies [8]. These supervised class-prediction studies were based on the idea that various molecular subgroups of breast cancer can be categorised by the aggregation of genes rather than individual genes. This approach involves the identification of a set of genes (a gene signature) that can be used collectively to identify tumours with specific biological or clinical features. The term 'genomic signatures' was used to refer to the expression of a set of genes in a biological sample using microarray technology, while the term 'metagene' refers to the aggregate measure of the expression of a group of genes that show coordinated expression in a set of samples. Most of these multigene assays were used in breast cancer to stratify prognostically clinically relevant groups into low and high risk subgroups to guide further treatment.

In addition to prognosis and prediction use, GEP technology has proved useful in other applications. For instance, microarray-based gene expression tests have been developed to identify the cancer tissue of origin. These include the Pathwork Tissue of Origin Test that was developed using a 2000-gene classification model for identification of tumour tissue of origin with an overall accuracy of up to 90% [9], and the THEROS Cancer TYPE ID which is a RT-PCR-based test that uses 92 genes and FFPE samples [10].

Although the clinical use of molecular classification of breast cancer remains limited, the introduction of the next generation sequencing (NGS) or massively parallel sequencing (MPS) [11] appears to open new avenues for decoding breast cancer molecular complexity, refining molecular classification and identifying new therapeutic targets. These techniques hold promise for improving diagnosis, prediction of outcome and behaviour, and in aiding selection of therapies for individual patients [12]. Circulating tumour cells (CTCs) have also received attention as biomarkers that may refine detection of metastatic disease and burden of metastatic tumour and monitor cancer progression. However, its clinical utility is still under investigation [13].

Although these molecular classification systems provide complimentary prognostic and improved predictive power than conventional variables, we still have a long way to go in terms of delivering truly personalised medicine. Here, we present a review of current and emerging molecular classification systems of breast cancer with emphasis on the molecular intrinsic subtype and multigene signatures.

MOLECULAR CLASSIFICATION OF BREAST CANCER USING INTRINSIC SUBTYPES

The first use of GEP to stratify breast cancer into molecularly distinct classes was introduced by Perou and colleagues in 2000 [3]. In their pioneering study, they demonstrated that breast cancer at the transcriptome level is not a single disease. Despite the fact that each individual tumour possesses a unique genetic profile, tumours clustered together to produce distinct reproducible classes based on transcriptomic profiles with common overlapping features that have biological and clinical significance.

The classification of breast cancer was based on the expression of a subset (n = 496) of differentially expressed genes termed the 'intrinsic' gene set. This intrinsic gene set was identified using a supervised analysis algorithm to select genes that show little variance within repeated samplings of the same tumour, but show high variance across tumours. Although no knowledge of outcome was used to derive this gene set, the distinct tumour subtypes identified showed prognostic significance.

In Perou's study [3], two main tumour clusters were identified according to their ER expression. The ER-positive cluster was enriched with ER, ER-related genes and other genes characteristic of the luminal epithelial cells, and this class was termed 'luminal' in reference to its molecular similarity to luminal mammary epithelial cells. The other cluster was ER-negative, and it exhibited three distinct subclasses, which were termed HER2-positive, basal-like and normal breast-like. The HER2 subgroup was characterised by overexpression of HER2 and other genes pertaining to HER2 amplicon. The basal-like class was largely characterised by the lack of expression of ER and HER2, by positive expression of genes characteristic of basal-like cells of the breast, and by a high proliferative activity. The normal breast-like class displayed a triple-negative phenotype, but it did not cluster with the basal-like centroid and was characterised by expression profiles similar to those found in normal breast tissue.

Importantly, these classes showed different clinical outcomes: the luminal subtype had the most favourable response whereas the HER2-positive class had the worst, and the basal-like subclass had a poor prognosis although it was relatively better than the HER2-positive, trastuzumab-naive cancers. Despite the identification of novel molecular classes and the prognostic significance of the 'intrinsic subtype' classification, this classification system showed strong concordance with the current classification systems that use ER, progesterone receptor (PR) and HER2, and the evidence for changing treatment of the few discordant cases based on intrinsic subtype remains insufficient. For instance, membership of the HER intrinsic subclass does not necessarily imply HER2 gene amplification and protein overexpression, and patients with HER2 gene amplified tumours remain candidates for anti-HER2 targeted therapy regardless of the intrinsic subtype of the tumour.

Subsequent GEP studies indicated that the luminal class, which comprises the majority of breast cancer, is heterogeneous with respect to the expression of other genes and outcome [14]. Many studies report at least two subclasses: luminal A and B subtypes. The former is identifiable by high levels of expression of ER and ER-activated genes, low levels of proliferation related genes, negative HER2 and having the best outcome. The luminal B class, on the other hand, was not clearly defined. Most studies indicate that luminal B tumours are associated with a worse prognosis, but the molecular definition was variable and not reproducible. In general, it was characterised by ER expression but with higher proliferation rates and/or HER2 expression and low or absent PR expression [15]. Other luminal subclasses have been described, for example luminal C [16] and luminal N [17], but luminal A and B remain the most validated subtypes despite its limitations.

Similarly to the luminal class, a number of studies have classified basal-like tumours into subgroups. In a study of 587 triple-negative breast cancers, Lehman and colleagues [18] reported six subtypes, each displaying a unique gene expression profile. These were basal-like I, basal-like II, an immunomodulatory, a mesenchymal, a mesenchymal stem-like and a luminal androgen receptor (AR) subtype. The differential response of these subtypes to neoadjuvant chemotherapy has been investigated [19]. Other studies report four subtypes of triple-negative breast cancer (luminal AR, mesenchymal, basal-like immune-suppressed and basal-like immune-activated) [20].

Despite the different microarray platforms and the different intrinsic gene lists which varied from several hundred to 1300 genes with limited overlap [21], most studies have consistently reported at least four classes, namely luminal A and B, HER2-positive and basal-like subtypes. Other novel molecular classes have also been described, such as the claudin-low subtype which exhibits reduced expression of genes involved in tight junctions and intercellular adhesion and increased expression of immune response genes [22]. This class is located using hierarchical clustering near the basal-like tumours, and both share some characteristic gene expression such as low expression of HER2 and luminal gene cluster. Other classes include the molecular apocrine subtype, characterised by the expression of androgen receptor and related genes. Both claudin-low and apocrine subtype have a triple-negative phenotype and a poor clinical outcome.

A genomics-driven classification of breast cancer based on an integrative analysis of GEP and genome-wide CNAs was reported by the Molecular Taxonomy of Breast Cancer International Consortium (METABRIC) [23]. This study of 2000 breast cancers reported that the number of molecular subtypes is likely to be 10, which are called 'integrative clusters', and that these subtypes showed distinct clinical behaviours. The METABRIC study also confirmed that triple-negative tumours are characterised by complex patterns of copy number gains and losses throughout the genome.

Although identification of these 10 integrative clusters was based on multiplatform molecular subtyping system using GEP and CNAs, in a subsequent study of 7544 breast cancers, Ali et al [24] reported that these integrative clusters can be identified by a gene-expression based approach alone, and that this classification system may be more informative in some contexts than the intrinsic subtype system. The Cancer Genome Atlas (TCGA) network [25] has analysed 466 breast cancers across five platforms: genomic DNA copy number arrays, DNA methylation, exome sequencing, mRNA arrays, microRNA sequencing and reverse phase protein arrays. The integrated findings (1) demonstrated the existence of four main breast cancer classes, (2) identified two novel protein expression defined subgroups related to stromal/micro-environmental elements and (3) provided key insights into previously defined gene expression subtypes. TCGA hypothesised that much of the clinically observable heterogeneity and plasticity occurs within, and not across, these major molecular subtypes. Research into molecular portraits of breast cancer is active, with many ongoing large scale studies utilising multiple platforms that will probably lead to further refinement of the molecular classification of breast cancer over the coming years.

To overcome the problems of fresh tissue, the availability of microarray-based technology, cost and assay reproducibility, other techniques such as RT-PCR and IHC coupled with tissue microarrays have been introduced to replicate this molecular taxonomy and to identify intrinsic subtypes in routine practice. Two approaches have been identified. The first involves the identification of a minimum gene set from microarray-based studies, which is then used to identify the GEP-defined classes. One successful example is the PAM50 (prediction of microarray using 50 classifier genes plus 5 reference genes) classifier [26]. PAM50 categorises breast cancer into the four intrinsic subtypes: luminal A, luminal B, HER2-enriched and basal-like, and it provides independent prognostic significance. It has been reported that a three-gene model, ESR1, ERBB2 and AURKA (SCMGENE), can also identify the four major breast cancer intrinsic subtypes. Although both classifiers provide independent prognostic information, other studies have reported that PAM50 provides greater prognostic information than the 3-genes SCMGENE assay and that the PAM50 assay but not the SCMGENE provides independent predictive information of pathological complete response in multivariate models. This may be explained by the greater amount of gene expression diversity of PAM50, and it also further supports the idea that identification of the major and clinically relevant molecular subtypes of breast cancer are best captured using larger gene panels [27].

The second approach for identifying intrinsic breast cancer subtypes in routine practice uses tissue microarrays and IHC. Utilising a large panel of biologically relevant biomarkers, these techniques apply unsupervised clustering techniques to identify molecular classes with and without comparison with GEP defined molecular subtypes. In a previous study, we applied 25 IHC biomarkers to 1950 unselected breast cancer series [28] and identified seven molecular classes. For practical reasons, we limited the number of genes used to identify those classes in routine practice to ten [17]. As the performance of clinicopathological factors varies among the seven molecular classes, the concept of refining the Nottingham Prognostic Index (NPI) applied equally to breast cancer regardless of the molecular features. NPI Plus (NPI+) was based on classifying breast cancer into seven distinct molecular classes using those ten biomarkers, after which we incorporated clinicopathological variables to identify distinct prognostic groups within each of the seven classes [29]. Using the NPI+ formulae, through incorporating molecular features and clinicopathological parameters, a patients' outcome stratification superior to the traditional NPI was achieved [29].

In a more simplified approach, some authors have used the three routinely available markers (ER, PR and HER2) plus KI67 to classify breast cancer into four molecular classes, with KI67 being used to stratify luminal tumours into two subclasses [2]. In a previous meta-analysis of more than 10,000 breast cancers, Blows et al [30] reported six intrinsic subtypes using five IHC markers (ER, PR, HER2, EGFR and CK5/6). In the recently published ESMO Clinical Practice guidelines, breast cancer is classified into five molecular subtypes based on the expression of those four markers with or without the addition of molecular gene signatures:

- Luminal A tumours are defined as ER- and PR-positive, HER2-negative, KI67 low (≤10%) and low-risk molecular signature (if available).
- Luminal B tumours are subclassified into luminal B HER2-positive and luminal HER2-negative but with either high proliferative activity (KI67 ≥ 30%), PR low or showing poor prognostic gene expression signature if available.
- Basal-like is defined as triple negative.
- HER2-positive is defined as HER2 overexpression/gene amplification with absence of ER and PR [31].

Similarly, the international expert panel at the St Gallen International Breast Cancer Conference in 2013 endorsed the use of PR expression in defining luminal A breast cancer for those cases having substantial PR expression (≥20%). They have also recommended a Ki67 threshold of ≥20% as an indicative of high Ki67 status in defining luminal B cancers [32].

However, it remains unknown how many molecular classes or intrinsic subtypes exist, and more importantly how many classes can be reliably identified with the currently available data and how accurate current molecular classification systems are. Thus, this molecular classification system remains a model in development.

MULTIGENE PROGNOSTIC AND PREDICTIVE SIGNATURES

In addition to intrinsic subtype classification, microarray-based GEP has been expanded to identify relevant classes (class prediction) using supervised clustering techniques. These class prediction GEP studies attempted to forecast outcomes for individual patients with breast cancer. This class prediction approach was pioneered by van't Veer et al [33] who selected a 70-gene signature based on the association of the expression of each gene with the likelihood of metastasis within 5 years. In summary, out of the 25,000 genes on the microarray, 5000 genes significantly regulated in >3 tumours were selected. Out of those 5000, 231 genes were found to correlate with outcome. Further refinement of the genes revealed that the minimum optimal marker genes that predict outcome were 70 genes. This 70-gene signature was validated on a group of 295 patients [33] and was later commercially marketed as MammaPrint assay (Agilent, Amsterdam, the Netherlands) (Table 2.1). The poor prognostic signature was characterised by up-regulation of genes involved in cell cycle, angiogenesis, signal transduction, proliferation, invasion and metastasis.

As the indications for adjuvant chemotherapy in breast cancer are more complex, a common application of gene signature assays is the identification of breast cancer patients with a sufficiently good prognosis that adjuvant chemotherapy can be safely omitted. Despite the effort invested in developing prognostic gene signatures, most signatures are reduced to two or three risk categories (i.e. low, intermediate and high). Chemotherapy is sufficient for patients with low-risk tumours, while those with high-risk tumours are candidates for such treatment. In clinical settings where adjuvant chemotherapy is indicated, gene signatures appeared less useful and omitting chemotherapy based on gene signatures in these circumstances require validation in large randomised trials.

The most frequent application of prognostic gene signatures in breast cancer remains in the clinical indeterminate group of ER-positive, HER2-negative and lymph node-negative or with low nodal burden disease. In fact, most studies have demonstrated that combining molecular signatures with the conventional factors provides the most useful prognostic information. Other gene signatures have been developed to predict the response to specific therapies.

Initial class prediction studies that attempted to identify gene signatures that predicted outcome were empirical, and based on profiling of tumours from patients with good or poor outcomes and collections of genes that discriminated between them [8]. Despite the minimal overlap between gene signatures and the fact that they were identified purely on their correlative and predictive value without consideration for the underlying mechanisms, most of them showed clinically significant risk stratification [41].

Although these first-generation gene signatures were composed of different gene lists, they mainly related to the expression of proliferation-associated genes. Given that the majority of ER-negative tumours have high expression levels of proliferation-related genes, these first generation signatures showed the highest discriminatory power in ER-positive disease. Subsequent studies have attempted to generate multigene predictors based on hypotheses derived from in vivo or in vitro experiments, or based on genes characteristic of a biological process [42,43]. Examples of the latter include genes associated with host immune responses, wound healing and other stromal gene signatures that carry prognostic value independent of ER status and proliferation [44]. Other gene signatures have been developed to classify breast cancer into subgroups based on response to specific therapies or prediction of outcome of patients treated with a particular type of therapy [45]. **Table 2.1** shows some of the most common gene signatures reported in breast cancer. Some examples are provided below.

MammaPrint score

MammaPrint is a microarray-based prognostic score that utilises fresh tissue or tissue that has been treated with a special solution. It is approved by the US Food and Drug Administration (FDA) for breast cancer patients >61 years with stage I/II, lymph node-negative or 1–3 node-positive disease and is performed by a central laboratory [4]. MammaPrint stratifies patients into low-risk or high-risk prognostic groups [33]. Although it is applicable to breast cancer regardless of ER expression, the prognostic risk discrimination is mainly seen in the ER-positive tumours, while ER-negative breast cancers are almost always classified as high risk, limiting its clinical value in ER-negative tumours. The MammaPrint test has been validated in retrospective studies, but its clinical utility is under investigation in a large prospective phase III trial: MINDACT (microarray in node-negative and 1–3 node-positive disease may avoid chemotherapy) that accrued 6600 patients between 2006 and 2011. Results are yet to be published.

Oncotype DX assay

The Oncotype DX is a RT-PCR-based assay performed on FFPE breast cancer samples. Oncotype DX uses 21 genes (16 cancer-related genes and 5 reference housekeeping genes) to compute a recurrence score from 0 to 100, which can be categorised into low risk (score <18), intermediate risk (score 18–30) or high risk (score ≥31) groups [34]. The Oncotype DX was developed for the purpose of splitting hormone therapy-treated patients who did not receive chemotherapy into two risk groups, and it has been validated in similar

Table 2.1 Prognostic and predictive gene signatures in early stage invasive breast cancer

Test name/vendor	Component gene(s)	Intended clinical utility	Biological material/ technology	Classification
Microarray and RT-PCR based assays				
Oncotype DX (recurrence score) (Genomic Health) [34]	21 genes (16 cancer-related and 5 controls)	ER+, HER2-, node-negative breast cancer. Predicts the likelihood of chemotherapy benefit as well as recurrence in hormone therapy treated patients. Test may extend to node-positive patients	FFPE, RT-PCR	3 categories: low risk (RS < 18), intermediate risk (RS 18–30), or high risk (RS > 31)
MammaPrint/ Amsterdam Signature (Agendia) [33]	70 genes (first prognostic gene signature to be identified)	Node-negative ER+ or ER− Estimates the recurrence risk. Test may extend to node positive patients	Fresh or FFPE, microarray	2 categories: low risk and high risk
Genomic Grade Index (GGI; MapQuant Dx) (Ipsogen)[35]	97 genes (related to tumour grade). A modified version using 8 genes and RT-PCR	Test can reclassify grade 2 ER+ breast cancer into high or low molecular grade	Fresh tissue (microarray) or FFPE (RT-PCR)	
Molecular grade index (MGI) (Biotheranostics) [36]	5 genes (proliferation related)	ER+ node-negative patients treated with hormone therapy.	FFPE, RT-PCR	2 categories: low and high risk of recurrence
Two-Gene Expression Ratio (H/I) (Quest Diagnostics) [36]	Ratio of the relative mRNA expression of 2 genes (HOXB13 : IL17BR)	ER-positive, node-negative patients	FFPE, RT-PCR	2 categories: low and high risk
THEROS Breast Cancer Index (BCI) (Biotheranostics) [36]	A combination of MGI (5 genes) and the 2 gene ratio (H/I) (HOXB13:IL17BR)	Risk of distant recurrence in ER+ node-negative breast cancer. Risk of late distant metastasis and benefit from extended (>5 years) endocrine therapy	FFPE, RT-PCR	
The Rotterdam Signature (Veridex) [37]	76 genes (60 genes for ER+ and 16 genes for ER- patients)	Node-negative patients. Predicts recurrence in ER+ treated with tamoxifen	Fresh tissue, microarray	
EndoPredict (Sividon Diagnostics) [38]	11 genes (8 cancer-related and 3 controls)	Predicts distant and late recurrences in ER+/HER2- node-negative and node-positive patients treated with endocrine therapy alone	FFPE, RT-PCR	Can be combined with tumour size and nodal status to produce clinical score

Table continued...

Table continued...

Test name/vendor	Component gene(s)	Intended clinical utility	Biological material/technology	Classification
Prosigna (PAM50) Kit (risk of recurrence assay; ROR) (NanoString Technologies) [39]	50 genes (used in the PAM50 molecular classification assay) and 5 control genes	ER+ node-negative and node-positive patients treated with hormone therapy. Evaluates distant recurrence-free survival at 10 years	FFPE, RT-PCR and by the nCounter Dx analysis system	3 categories: low, intermediate and high risk
BreastOncPx (Lab Corp)	14 genes (not including ER or HER2)	Risk of distant metastasis (metastasis score). Helps identify higher-risk patients who might benefit from additional therapy	FFPE, RT-PCR	
Celera Metastasis Score (Lab Corp)	14 genes	ER+, node-negative patients treated with hormone therapy	FFPE, RT-PCR	2 categories: low and high risk
Invasiveness Gene Signature (IGS) (OncoMed Pharmaceuticals) [38b]	186 genes	Both ER and node-positive and node-negative patients	Fresh tissue, microarray	
Immunohistochemistry (IHC) and in situ hybridisation (ISH)-based tests				
IHC4 score [39]	4 genes (ER, PR, Ki67 and HER2)	ER+ patients treated with hormone therapy	FFPE and IHC	
Insight Dx Mammostrat (Clarient Diagnostic Services)	5 genes	ER+, node-negative patients treated with tamoxifen alone Predicts benefit from additional cytotoxic chemotherapy	FFPE and IHC	3 categories: low, intermediate and high
Insight Dx Mammostrat Plus (Clarient Diagnostic Services)	9 genes (As above plus ER, PR, KI67 and HER2)	As above, plus hormone receptor/HER2 status	FFPE, additional genes evaluated by IHC and FISH	2 categories
ProEx Br (The BD/TriPath)	5 genes (5 antibody /5 separate slide IHC assay that uses an image analysis system)	Overexpression of ≥2 markers (score ≥2) has been associated with disease relapse in node-negative and node-positive patients	FFPE, IHC	2 categories
eXagenBC (eXagen Diagnostics)	3 genes (DNA Copy number) for ER-positive and 3 genes for ER-negative tumours	Node-negative and node-positive patients	FFPE and FISH	2 categories: low and high risk
Signatures based on a biological process				
Wound-response signature [40]	442 genes	Node-negative and node-positive patients	Fresh, microarray	2 categories
Immune signatures	14 genes related to immune function	Predictive for relapse in trastuzumab-treated HER2+ patients		2 categories
Invasiveness Gene Signature (IGS)	186 genes	Predicts 10-year distant metastasis free survival in node-negative patients	Fresh, microarray	2 categories

FFPE, formalin-fixed paraffin-embedded; ER, oestrogen receptor; PR, progesterone receptor; RT-PCR, reverse transcription-polymerase chain reaction; FISH, fluorescence in situ hybridisation.

independent studies. These studies indicated that the Oncotype DX score predicts the likelihood of distant recurrence or breast cancer death in ER-positive patients treated with hormonal therapy alone and demonstrated benefit from adjuvant chemotherapy primarily in patients with high recurrence score. Currently, Oncotype DX is the most widely used prognostic assay for ER-positive node-negative breast cancer in the UK and the USA. The clinical utility of Oncotype DX is currently under further investigation in large prospective randomised clinical trials: TAILORx (patients with ER+, HER2–, node-negative breast cancer) and RxPONDER [patients with ER+, HER2– breast cancer with 1–3 positive nodes (N1)].

PAM50 risk of recurrence score (Prosigna kit)

Although PAM50 test was developed to identify breast cancer molecular intrinsic subtypes using FFPE tissue on a RT-PCR platform, the assay has been modified into a simple molecular test for predicting outcome by generating a numerical risk score (abbreviated to 'ROR', or risk of recurrence) which parallels that of Oncotype DX [39]. The PAM50 ROR assay has been adopted as the 'Prosigna Breast Cancer Prognostic Gene Signature' by a commercial partner (Nanostring Technologies, Seattle, WA, USA). The Prosigna assay utilises the nanotechnology-based nCounter digital gene expression platform, allowing it to be performed in any pathology laboratory. The Prosigna kit quantifies mRNA expression of 50 genes used in the PAM50 molecular classification algorithm and 5 housekeeping genes and computes the ROR, which reflects the intrinsic breast cancer subtype of the case. Prosigna can be used to estimate short- and long-term recurrence-free survival for stage I/II (including 1–3 positive nodes) ER-positive breast cancer in postmenopausal women treated with adjuvant hormone therapy [39]. The Prosigna Kit was approved by FDA and has received clearance in the EU. Prosigna has also been selected as the genomic test in the OPTIMA main trial, which follows on from the preliminary phase of this study, OPTIMA prelim. The OPTIMA prelim study used a five-multigene genomic test and included 301 patients. OPTIMA (Optimal Personalised Treatment of early breast cancer using Multi-parameter Analysis) is a UK-based clinical trial that aims to reduce the use of chemotherapy in hormone response HER2-negative breast cancer patients with lymph node-positive status (pN1-2 or pN0 and pT > 30 mm) who are currently offered chemotherapy as standard treatment [46].

Breast cancer index

Breast cancer index (BCI) consists of two independently developed gene signatures: molecular grade index (MGI), a five-gene predictor that recapitulates tumour grade/proliferation; and the two-gene ratio (*HOXB13/IL17BR*) signature (H/I), which was developed independent of tumour grade/proliferation. Compared to Oncotype DX and IHC4, BCI is a predictor of early distant recurrence and is the only significant prognostic for risk of late recurrence [47].

EndoPredict

The EndoPredict test (Sividon Diagnostics GmbH, Koln, Germany) is an RT-PCR-based assay using FFPE tissue, and it measures the expression of eight breast cancer-related genes and three housekeeping genes. It stratifies ER-positive breast cancer patients treated with adjuvant endocrine therapy alone into low or high risk of recurrence. The EndoPredict score has also been combined with clinical variables, namely lymph node stage and tumour size, to compute a clinical risk score termed EPclin that shows predictive value for identification of ER-positive patients at risk for late recurrence [48]. The assay is marketed in Germany and Europe as a prognostic kit that can be performed by local laboratories.

IHC4 assay

The IHC4 assay uses IHC and FFPE tissue and is based on the assessment of ER, PR, HER2 and Ki67. It takes the semiquantitative expression values of these four markers and produces a ROR score.

IHC4 has provided prognostic stratification comparable to the other costly multigene signatures such as Oncotype DX. Although IHC4 is inexpensive and can be performed in local laboratories, standardisation of IHC4 and quality assurance programs are required before its use becomes widespread [39].

Most currently available multigene signature assays provide significant independent prognostic value in ER-positive HER2-negative breast cancer, particularly in the node-negative or low burden disease. Although comparative studies of these molecular assays indicate that discordant risk prediction occurs when different prognostic assays are applied to the same tumour, each provide independent prognostic signature when considered alone. In a previous study, six-gene signature assays, including Oncotype DX, PAM50/ROR and MammaPrint, were applied to the same patient cohort, and although each test provided significant prognostic value, individual risk assignments were not often concordant [49], therefore the authors suggested that combining several multigene tests may offer more accurate outcome prediction [49].

Although most gene signatures available have little or no prognostic value in HER2-positive and ER-negative tumours, some studies have reported prognostic stratification power for specific sets of genes. For instance, a prognostic predictor based on 158 genes [HER2-derived prognostic predictor (HDPP)] has been found to provide more accurate stratification of tumours into good and bad prognosis [50]. Similarly, prognostic signatures linked to genes involved in immune, inflammatory and/or chemokine pathways have been developed for ER-negative breast cancer. GEP has also been used to subdivide triple-negative breast cancer into distinct groups, and a prognostic significance of a ratio of B-cell and interleukin-8 (IL-8) metagenes has provided a prognosis value in triple-negative disease. Although there is a near consensus that multigene prognostic assays provide useful complementary information to well-established traditional clinicopathological variables in ER-positive tumours, it is not surprising that clinically useful prognostic signatures for HER2 positive ER-negative breast cancer are still non-existent.

NEXT GENERATION SEQUENCING

NGS has revolutionised breast cancer genetics and genomics, and it is expected to pave the path for personalised treatment of breast cancer patients. Common uses of NGS include whole-genome sequencing, whole-exome sequencing, targeted exome sequencing (target-enrichment methods to capture genes of interest) and hotspot (sequences selected regions/regions with recurrent mutations of selected genes of interest) sequencing. NGS has been used to characterise genomic alterations such as copy number changes, insertions/deletions and mutations; to facilitate sequencing at a greater depth (at the base-pair level); to enable the identification of subclonal mutations; and to help differentiate 'driver' mutations that contribute to cancer development from 'passenger' mutations that do not appear to play a significant role in cancer development.

In addition to providing information about the genomic landscape of breast cancer, NGS has confirmed both intertumour and intratumour heterogeneity and showed that each breast cancer is largely unique.

NGS has been used to show that mutation frequencies in breast cancer are lower than in other cancers, such as lung squamous cell carcinoma or bladder urothelial carcinomas, but are similar to those of ovarian and renal clear cell carcinomas. In a NGS study of 100 breast cancers [51], the number of somatic mutations was reported to vary markedly between individual tumours, and to correlate with patient age and histological grade. Multiple mutational signatures were observed and driver mutations were identified in at least 40 cancer genes including new cancer genes [51]. Somatic driver point mutations and/or copy number changes were identified in at least 40 cancer genes. There was a maximum of 6 mutated cancer genes in an individual breast cancer, and 28 cases of the 100 showed a single driver. Seven of those 40 cancer genes (TP53, PIK3CA, MYC, ERBB2, FGFR1, CCND1 and GATA3) were mutated in >10% of cases and these contributed 58% of driver mutations [51]. Overall, the study sample had a mean of 56.9 (range 5–374) somatic mutations per cancer.

TCGA network reported different genetic abnormalities associated with the molecular intrinsic subtypes. 40% of luminal A tumours had a mutated PIK3CA gene. PIK3CA and TP53 were mutated in 29% of luminal B tumours. TP53 was mutated in 80% of basal-like classes which exhibited a more consistent pattern and the highest amount of mutations compared to luminal tumours. The HER2-enriched tumours showed HER2 amplification in 80% of cases [25]. The vast majority (76%) of breast cancers are characterised and driven by recurrent CAN (C class), while tumours characterised and driven by recurrent mutations (M class) are almost exclusively of luminal subtype (92%), and 99% of basal-like tumours are of C class [52].

NGS has also been used to demonstrate the spatial and temporal intratumour heterogeneity of breast cancer. Various degrees of intratumour genetic heterogeneity have been found, even in the absence of overt histological phenotypic heterogeneity. Triple-negative and basal-like tumours tend to have greater intratumour heterogeneity than nonbasal-like tumours. Mutations in common driver genes such as TP53, PIK3CA and PTEN are usually found in high clonal frequencies and several somatic mutations are present in only a fraction of cancer cells. NGS also showed that the constellations of somatic mutations found between a primary breast cancer and its metastases (temporal heterogeneity) and between distinct areas within the primary tumour (spatial heterogeneity) are not identical providing further evidence to indicate that breast cancer evolve over the course of the disease. This clonal genetic heterogeneity may explain resistance of some breast cancer to selective environmental pressures and therapy.

CONCLUSION

Molecular testing is becoming increasingly important in the prevention, diagnosis and treatment of breast cancer. Despite the enormous amount of work that has been carried out to develop and refine breast cancer molecular classification, it is still evolving. With the increasing use of more sophisticated high-throughput techniques such as MPS, large amounts of data will continue to emerge, which may lead to the identification of novel therapeutic targets and provide the basis for more precise classification systems.

Key points for clinical practice

- Breast cancer is a diverse spectrum of diseases featuring distinct histological, biological, molecular and clinical phenotypes.

- Studies indicate that traditional classification systems are insufficient to reflect the biological and clinical heterogeneity of breast cancer because tumours of similar clinicopathological features exhibit dissimilar behaviour and responses to specific therapy, but advances in high-throughput molecular techniques and bioinformatics have improved our understanding of breast cancer biology, refined molecular taxonomies and led to the development of novel prognostic and predictive molecular assays.

- Molecular testing is becoming relevant to the prevention, diagnosis and treatment of breast cancer. Molecular prognostic and predictive assays are still evolving, but there are only a small number relevant to routine clinical practice and these are focussed on identifying patients at high risk of relapse, or patients who have potential to benefit from adjuvant chemotherapy in the context of lymph node negative, oestrogen receptor positive breast cancer.

- With the increasing use of more sophisticated molecular techniques, such as next generation sequencing, novel therapeutic targets will be identified, and also to support more precise classification systems.

REFERENCES

1. Rakha EA, Reis-Filho JS, Baehner F, et al. Breast cancer prognostic classification in the molecular era: the role of histological grade. Breast Cancer Res 2010; 12:207.
2. Aleskandarany MA, Green AR, Benhasouna AA, et al. Prognostic value of proliferation assay in the luminal, HER2-positive, and triple-negative biologic classes of breast cancer. Breast Cancer Res 2012; 14:R3.
3. Perou CM, Sorlie T, Eisen MB, et al. Molecular portraits of human breast tumours. Nature 2000; 406:747–752.
4. Sorlie T, Perou CM, Tibshirani R, et al. Gene expression patterns of breast carcinomas distinguish tumor subclasses with clinical implications. Proc Natl Acad Sci USA 2001; 98:10869–10874.
5. Davies C, Godwin J, Gray R, et al. Relevance of breast cancer hormone receptors and other factors to the efficacy of adjuvant tamoxifen: patient-level meta-analysis of randomised trials. Lancet 2011; 378:771–784.
6. Early Breast Cancer Trialists' Collaborative Group. Effects of chemotherapy and hormonal therapy for early breast cancer on recurrence and 15-year survival: an overview of the randomised trials. Lancet 2005; 365:1687–1717.
7. Bastien RR, Rodriguez-Lescure A, Ebbert MT, et al. PAM50 breast cancer subtyping by RT-qPCR and concordance with standard clinical molecular markers. BMC Medical Genomics 2012; 5:44.
8. van't Veer LJ, Dai H, van de Vijver MJ, et al. Gene expression profiling predicts clinical outcome of breast cancer. Nature 2002; 415:530–536.
9. Monzon FA, Lyons-Weiler M, Buturovic LJ, et al. Multicenter validation of a 1,550-gene expression profile for identification of tumor tissue of origin. J Clin Oncol 2009; 27:2503–2508.
10. Ma XJ, Patel R, Wang X, et al. Molecular classification of human cancers using a 92-gene real-time quantitative polymerase chain reaction assay. Arch Pathol Lab Med 2006; 130:465–473.
11. Torres TT, Metta M, Ottenwalder B, et al. Gene expression profiling by massively parallel sequencing. Genome Res 2008; 18:172–177.
12. Ng CK, Schultheis AM, Bidard FC, et al. Breast cancer genomics from microarrays to massively parallel sequencing: paradigms and new insights. J Natl Cancer Inst 2015; 107 (5) doi: 10.1093/jnci/djv015.
13. Alix-Panabieres C, Pantel K. Challenges in circulating tumour cell research. Nat Rev Cancer 2014; 14:623–631.
14. Sorlie T, Tibshirani R, Parker J, et al. Repeated observation of breast tumor subtypes in independent gene expression data sets. Proc Natl Acad Sci U S A 2003; 100:8418–8423.

15. Habashy HO, Powe DG, Abdel-Fatah TM, et al. A review of the biological and clinical characteristics of luminal-like oestrogen receptor-positive breast cancer. Histopathology 2012; 60:854–863.
16. Sotiriou C, Neo SY, McShane LM, et al. Breast cancer classification and prognosis based on gene expression profiles from a population-based study. Proc Natl Acad Sci U S A 2003; 100:10393–10398.
17. Rakha EA, Soria D, Green AR, et al. Nottingham Prognostic Index Plus (NPI+): a modern clinical decision making tool in breast cancer. Br J Cancer 2014; 110:1688–1697.
18. Lehmann BD, Bauer JA, Chen X, et al. Identification of human triple-negative breast cancer subtypes and preclinical models for selection of targeted therapies. J Clin Invest 2011; 121:2750–2767.
19. Masuda H, Baggerly KA, Wang Y, et al. Differential response to neoadjuvant chemotherapy among 7 triple-negative breast cancer molecular subtypes. Clin Cancer Res 2013; 19:5533–5540.
20. Burstein MD, Tsimelzon A, Poage GM, et al. Comprehensive genomic analysis identifies novel subtypes and targets of triple-negative breast cancer. Clin Cancer Res 2015; 21:1688–1698.
21. Hu Z, Fan C, Oh DS, et al. The molecular portraits of breast tumors are conserved across microarray platforms. BMC Genomics 2006; 7:96.
22. Prat A, Parker JS, Karginova O, et al. Phenotypic and molecular characterisation of the claudin-low intrinsic subtype of breast cancer. Breast Cancer Res 2010; 12:R68.
23. Curtis C, Shah SP, Chin SF, et al. The genomic and transcriptomic architecture of 2,000 breast tumours reveals novel subgroups. Nature 2012; 486:346–352.
24. Ali HR, Rueda OM, Chin SF, et al. Genome-driven integrated classification of breast cancer validated in over 7,500 samples. Genome Biol 2014; 15:431.
25. Cancer Genome Atlas N. Comprehensive molecular portraits of human breast tumours. Nature 2012; 490:61–70.
26. Parker JS, Mullins M, Cheang MC, et al. Supervised risk predictor of breast cancer based on intrinsic subtypes. J Clin Oncol 2009; 27:1160–1167.
27. Prat A, Parker JS, Fan C, et al. PAM50 assay and the three-gene model for identifying the major and clinically relevant molecular subtypes of breast cancer. Breast Cancer Res Treat 2012; 135:301–306.
28. Abd El-Rehim DM, Ball G, Pinder SE, et al. High-throughput protein expression analysis using tissue microarray technology of a large well-characterised series identifies biologically distinct classes of breast cancer confirming recent cDNA expression analyses. Int J Cancer 2005; 116:340–350.
29. Rakha EA, Soria D, Green AR, et al. Nottingham Prognostic Index Plus (NPI+): a modern clinical decision making tool in breast cancer. BMJ 2014; 110:1688–1697.
30. Blows FM, Driver KE, Schmidt MK, et al. Subtyping of breast cancer by immunohistochemistry to investigate a relationship between subtype and short and long term survival: a collaborative analysis of data for 10,159 cases from 12 studies. PLoS Med 2010; 7:e1000279.
31. Senkus E, Kyriakides S, Ohno S, et al. Primary breast cancer: ESMO Clinical Practice Guidelines for diagnosis, treatment and follow-up. Ann Oncol 2015; 26:v8–v30.
32. Goldhirsch A, Winer EP, Coates AS, et al. Personalising the treatment of women with early breast cancer: highlights of the St Gallen International Expert Consensus on the Primary Therapy of Early Breast Cancer 2013. Ann Oncol 2013; 24:2206–2223.
33. van de Vijver MJ, He YD, van't Veer LJ, et al. A gene-expression signature as a predictor of survival in breast cancer. N Engl J Med 2002; 347:1999–2009.
34. Paik S, Shak S, Tang G, et al. A multigene assay to predict recurrence of tamoxifen-treated, node-negative breast cancer. N Engl J Med 2004; 351:2817–2826.
35. Toussaint J, Sieuwerts AM, Haibe-Kains B, et al. Improvement of the clinical applicability of the Genomic Grade Index through a qRT-PCR test performed on frozen and formalin-fixed paraffin-embedded tissues. BMC Genomics 2009; 10:424.
36. Ma XJ, Salunga R, Dahiya S, et al. A five-gene molecular grade index and HOXB13:IL17BR are complementary prognostic factors in early stage breast cancer. Clin Cancer Res 2008; 14:2601–2608.
37. Wang Y, Klijn JG, Zhang Y, et al. Gene-expression profiles to predict distant metastasis of lymph-node-negative primary breast cancer. Lancet 2005; 365:671–679.
38. Filipits M, Rudas M, Jakesz R, et al. A new molecular predictor of distant recurrence in ER-positive, HER2-negative breast cancer adds independent information to conventional clinical risk factors. Clin Cancer Res 2011; 17:6012–6020.
38b. Liu R, Wang X, Chen GY, et al. The prognostic role of a gene signature from tumorigenic breast-cancer cells. N Engl J Med 2007; 356:217–226.

39. Dowsett M, Sestak I, Lopez-Knowles E, et al. Comparison of PAM50 risk of recurrence score with oncotype DX and IHC4 for predicting risk of distant recurrence after endocrine therapy. J Clin Oncol 2013; 31:2783–2790.
40. Chang HY, Nuyten DS, Sneddon JB, et al. Robustness, scalability, and integration of a wound-response gene expression signature in predicting breast cancer survival. Proc Natl Acad Sci USA 2005; 102:3738–3743.
41. Kelly CM, Bernard PS, Krishnamurthy S, et al. Agreement in risk prediction between the 21-gene recurrence score assay (Oncotype DX(R)) and the PAM50 breast cancer intrinsic classifier in early-stage estrogen receptor-positive breast cancer. Oncologist 2012; 17:492–498.
42. Sotiriou C, Wirapati P, Loi S, et al. Gene expression profiling in breast cancer: understanding the molecular basis of histologic grade to improve prognosis. J Natl Cancer Inst 2006; 98:262–272.
43. Teschendorff AE, Miremadi A, Pinder SE, et al. An immune response gene expression module identifies a good prognosis subtype in estrogen receptor negative breast cancer. Genome Biol 2007; 8:R157.
44. Winslow S, Leandersson K, Edsjo A, et al. Prognostic stromal gene signatures in breast cancer. Breast Cancer Res 2015; 17:23.
45. Bonnefoi H, Potti A, Delorenzi M, et al. Validation of gene signatures that predict the response of breast cancer to neoadjuvant chemotherapy: a substudy of the EORTC 10994/BIG 00-01 clinical trial. Lancet Oncol 2007; 8:1071–1078.
46. Bartlett J, Canney P, Campbell A, et al. Selecting breast cancer patients for chemotherapy: the opening of the UK OPTIMA trial. Clin Oncol (R Coll Radiol) 2013; 25:109–116.
47. Sgroi DC, Sestak I, Cuzick J, et al. Prediction of late distant recurrence in patients with oestrogen-receptor-positive breast cancer: a prospective comparison of the breast-cancer index (BCI) assay, 21-gene recurrence score, and IHC4 in the TransATAC study population. Lancet Oncol 2013; 14:1067–1076.
48. Muller BM, Keil E, Lehmann A, et al. The EndoPredict Gene-Expression Assay in Clinical Practice – Performance and Impact on Clinical Decisions. PLoS One 2013; 8:e68252.
49. Prat A, Parker JS, Fan C, et al. Concordance among gene expression-based predictors for ER-positive breast cancer treated with adjuvant tamoxifen. Ann Oncol 2012; 23:2866–2873.
50. Staaf J, Ringner M, Vallon-Christersson J, et al. Identification of subtypes in human epidermal growth factor receptor 2 – positive breast cancer reveals a gene signature prognostic of outcome. J Clin Oncol 2010; 28:1813–1820.
51. Stephens PJ, Tarpey PS, Davies H, et al. The landscape of cancer genes and mutational processes in breast cancer. Nature 2012; 486:400–404.
52. Ciriello G, Miller ML, Aksoy BA, et al. Emerging landscape of oncogenic signatures across human cancers. Nat Genet 2013; 45:1127–1133.

Chapter 3

Genetic origins of human cancer

Trevor A Graham, Nicholas A Wright

INTRODUCTION

We usually credit Boveri for the first proposals concerning the role of somatic genetic changes in cancer progression [1], although Tyzzer [2] was perhaps the first to use the term 'somatic mutation' to designate events occurring in cancer progression. Though Armitage and Doll [3] sketched the stages of multistage progression from somatic mutations it was not until Knudson's [4] seminal studies, followed by the cloning of the *Rb* (retinoblastoma) gene, other tumour suppressor genes and oncogenes that Fearon and Vogelstein [5], analysing colorectal tumour progression, provided support for the proposal that cancer progresses through multiple stages, accompanied by changes in critical genes that drive progression – the multistep cancer progression model.

In this chapter, we shall discuss the reasons why this multistep theory, in its original form, no longer fits the data now available from studies of cancer development in humans, and discuss alternative models that might be more appropriate.

THE MULTISTEP CANCER PROGRESSION MODEL

The multistep cancer progression model, where tumours progressively accumulate carcinogenic mutations or other genetic changes, has held sway for many years [5,6]. These alterations often involve tumour suppressor genes and oncogenes, and occur in a stepwise fashion. This concept highlights the putative importance of the accumulation of genetic changes, and emphasises the order in which they occur; it is probably true to say that the concept of multistep cancer progression model has provided the basis for our understanding of the initiation, growth, progression and metastatic spread of cancer. Originally formulated for the progression of colorectal cancer, it has become the paradigm for thinking about tumour progression in a variety of other cancer sites (e.g. pancreas [7] and breast [8]). During this progressive clonal evolution [9], selectively advantageous 'driver' lesions [10] lead to the acquisition of the phenotypic 'hallmarks of cancer'- sustained proliferation, evading growth suppression and cell death, enabling replicative immortality, angiogenesis, and eventually invasion and metastasis [11,12].

Trevor A Graham PhD Centre for Tumour Biology, Barts Cancer Institute, Barts and the London School of Medicine and Dentistry, Queen Mary University of London, London UK. Email: t.graham@qmul.ac.uk (for correspondence)

Nicholas A Wright MA MD PhD DSc FRCPath Centre for Tumour Biology, Barts Cancer Institute, Barts and the London School of Medicine and Dentistry, Queen Mary University of London, London UK. Email: n.a.wright@qmul.ac.uk (for correspondence)

This model of tumour development is shown in **Figure 3.1**: a mutation occurs in a cell – possibly a stem cell [13] – which is selected and leads to a clonal expansion of these cells. A further mutation occurs, which is again selected to clonally expan,d replacing the other cells in the population – this is called a selective sweep [14]. When all cells in the population bear the mutation, the mutation is said to have 'swept to fixation' within the population. There follows a series of selective sweeps, until the malignant phenotype is reached. The whole preneoplastic (or neoplastic) population therefore always share a common ancestor more recent than the founder cell of the neoplastic lesion. This series of selective sweeps was to the best of our knowledge first proposed as a popular model for Barrett's oesophagus [15], a premalignant neoplastic condition of the oesophagus and an accepted precursor of oesophageal adenocarcinoma. In this condition, the normal oesophageal stratified squamous epithelium is replaced by a columnar epithelium that often shows intestinal differentiation [16] and is thought to develop as a complication of chronic reflux disease. In a large corpus of work from the Reid group in Seattle, patients with Barrett's oesophagus were followed longitudinally over a number of years with serial biopsies and the distribution of a number of mutations, notably $p16$ ($CDKN2A^{INK4A}$) and $p53$ ($TP53$). The spread of these mutations was documented with time after diagnosis, and it appeared that genetic lesions involving these genes could be detected over large regions of Barrett's epithelium. Moreover, the spread of these mutations could be rapid, with mutant clones growing through large areas of the Barrett's segment and the same clone can occupy as much as 17 cm of the segment. The spread of these mutations was often ascribed to fission of Barrett's glands [15].

This attractive model was also elegantly applied to colorectal tumourigenesis, similarly thought to proceed through morphologically defined stages each associated with distinctive mutations [5,17]. Most colorectal carcinomas arise through the adenoma/carcinoma sequence, where the adenoma – a localised collection of neoplastic tubules – is confined to the superficial part of the colon and does not invade. By comparing the mutation burden of tumours from each morphological stage, a single colorectal epithelial cell was envisaged as acquiring a mutation that inactivates the adenomatous polyposis coli (APC)/β-catenin (wnt) pathway, followed by waves of clonal expansion driven by

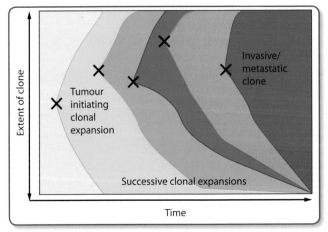

Figure 3.1 The sequential model of cancer progression. An initial mutation (black cross) that confers a selective advantage is acquired by a cell, and causes a clonal sweep. This first cell is probably a stem cell. Subsequent mutations in key driver genes (black crosses) to cells within this clone trigger subsequent clonal expansions, and each clone takes over the entire neoplasm (a sweep to fixation). The accrual of driver mutations in this stepwise fashion underpins the progression to an invasive or metastatic phenotype. In the colon, the canonical genetic model involves sequential mutations in the APC, KRAS and TP53 genes [5,6], whereas in Barrett's early mutation of p16 it is followed by later inactivation of TP53 [14].

mutations in *KRAS/BRAF*, *TGFβ*, *PIK3CA* and finally *TP53*. A word of caution here: computational modelling shows that this kind of 'cross-sectional' approach to inferring mutation order tends to misrepresent the order of mutations in any individual cancer [18], so at best this envisaged order can be interpreted only as the typical, but not requisite, order of somatic mutations. The carcinogenic process was described by assuming that that all somatic mutations occurred *clonally* in an adenoma – present in all its cells, but beginning with the cell of origin or founder cell: again probably a stem cell [19]. These mutations thus accumulate within the adenoma by a similar wave of selective sweeps, which go to fixation throughout the adenoma. It follows that adenomas should be 'genetically homogeneous benign lesion(s)' [20].

In summary, the multistep cancer progression is a model of the clonal evolution of a cancer that postulates that the cancer-causing 'driver' mutations accrue in a preferential order and each bestows a large selective advantage to the cell that acquires them, which is sufficient to drive the expansion of that clone to fixation in the cancer (**Figure 3.1**).

PROBLEMS WITH THE CLASSICAL MULTISTEP CANCER PROGRESSION MODEL

There are significant drawbacks to this model. In the first place, it suggests that there has to be an order in which mutations occur; elaborate schemes have been set out for the order in which mutations occur in a number of tumours. Clinically, a model postulating time-dependent series of mutations in the progression of cancer is appealing, because if tumour cells 'bottleneck' through a series of definitive steps, these might be amenable to therapeutic attack [21] or be useful 'milestones' that can be used for prognostication. For example, in the progression of Barrett's oesophagus, deletion at the *p16* locus occurs early and loss of *TP53* usually occurs after loss of *p16* [14]; thus, the presence of *TP53* lesion should be a maker of a Barrett's lesion that is closer to becoming cancerous. However, such a deterministic and reproducible progression through sequential mutations with a fixed order of selection is unlikely. It is more probable that tumours develop through variable pathways, and that the order of mutation/selection is mainly stochastic [21]. Nevertheless, it is clear that epistasis between mutated genes and tissue-specific interactions (e.g. the microenvironmental context) plays an important role in the selection for mutant genes [22]. Tellingly though, many driver mutations are detected in ostensibly 'normal' tissue, notably *p53* and oncogene mutations in both skin [23] and nondysplastic colon epithelium in inflammatory bowel disease [24].

Secondly, selective sweeps are rare in human tumours. In Barrett's oesophagus, a study that analysed the mutations in individual Barrett's glands from oesophagectomy specimens from Barrett's patients, rather than whole-biopsy DNA extracts, found no evidence of a founder mutation and instead supported the concept of small, localised clonal expansions. In fact, earlier studies had recognised that such mosaicism was often present [21]. More recently, a detailed longitudinal study of genetic progression in Barrett's patients with and without nonsteroidal anti-inflammatory drug (NSAID) treatment using genome-wide single nucleotide polymorphism (SNP) arrays showed that multiple clones coexist throughout the follow-up period [25]. In fact, in only one case, a clone grew to dominate the Barrett's segment over some 153 patient-years of follow-up, without real evidence that the clone swept to fixation. There was one patient who progressed to carcinoma and even here the clone that developed huge somatic genomic abnormalities was spatially restricted. A larger patient series confirmed this result [26].

Similar spatial localisation of 'driver' mutations has been reported in colorectal adenomas. **Figure 3.2** shows that, in human colorectal adenomas progressing to carcinomas, there are no selective sweeps. Instead, the adenoma itself is far from genetically homogenous, but has a complex structure, being composed of small clones, or subclones [27,28]. While intratumoural clones can indeed form near the inception of neoplasia, they do not sweep through the adenoma and appear as spatially localised clones, while rare subclones appear later in the development of the adenoma, occupying only focal regions of the tumour. Just by examining a few genes known to be mutated in colorectal cancer, it can be seen that adenomas show a complex regional genetic structure, with segregated clones that correlate with the histological appearances (**Figure 3.2**).

Indeed, the recent interest in intratumour heterogeneity, coupled with the recent availability of genome-wide analysis methods, makes it clear that genetic mosaicism is a feature of most, if not all, cancers [29]. For example, in kidney cancer, different regions of the same cancer contain different driver mutations [30,31] and evolving mutational processes characterise the evolution of lung cancer, although interestingly most driver mutations appeared on the trunk of phylogenetic trees [32,33]. Examples of intratumour heterogeneity in other tumour types include but are not limited to breast [34–36], glioma [37,38], leukaemia [39] and ovary [40]. Genetic heterogeneity over time is observed as well; genetic differences are observed between lymphomas at presentation and after progression [41] and in relapsing leukaemia [42]. As might be expected, genetic differences are observed between primary tumour and associated metastases [43] and phylogenetic analysis of these data reveals how metastases spread around the body [44]. The apparent ubiquity of genetic heterogeneity across cancers leads to questions about the frequencies of large-scale clonal sweeps to fixation in all cancer types.

From this brief survey, it is clear that the assumptions implicit in the classical multistep cancer progression model – that mutations sequentially spread throughout the tumour, creating a genetically homogeneous lesion in which all cells share the same mutations – are inconsistent with the data currently available.

The main hurdle in understanding the dynamics of human tumour growth is that we cannot directly witness tumour development because longitudinal surveillance is impractical. But what can we learn from single time point 'snapshots' of the clonal architecture of a tumour? Insightful mathematical analysis of clone size data from carcinogen-induced murine skin carcinomas has revealed that subclones within a tumour grow but also shrink over time, and, in fact, follow a process of neutral drift whereby the expansion or contraction of a clone over time is equally likely [45]. In this model system at least, the expansion of subclones within a tumour is an inherently stochastic process where the clonal composition is ever changing in a somewhat unpredictable way. In the intestine, quantitative analysis of clonal expansions showed that clones bearing (transgenically induced) mutations in the important drivers *KRAS*, *APC* or *TP53* followed stochastic, not deterministic, patterns of growth which meant that sometimes these driver mutations were driven extinct through competition with the resident (but less fit) population of wild-type cells in the crypt [46]. Although detailed quantitation of the expansions of clones bearing driver mutations has not been performed in human tissues, similar stochastic clonal expansion dynamics are consistent with that available in intestinal adenomas [28,47] and morphologically normal lung from cancer patients [48]. These studies demonstrate that in the cases where measurements have been performed, subclones do not expand deterministically within tumours. Instead, chance plays a big role in the deciding the

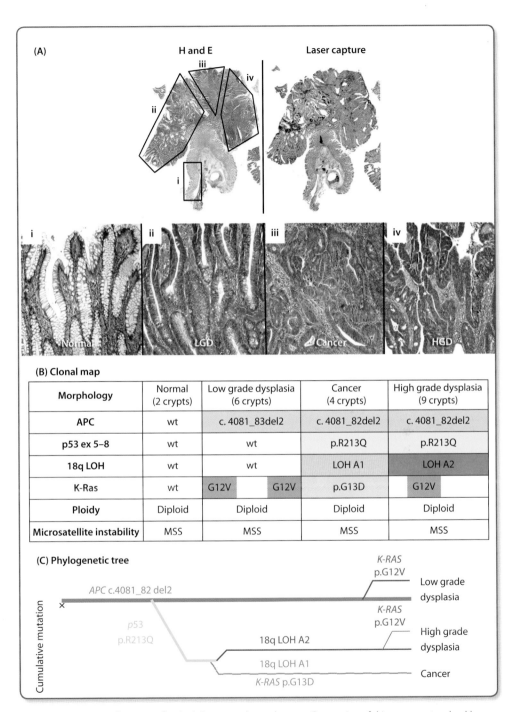

Figure 3.2 Genetic architecture of an 'early' human colorectal cancer. Genotyping of driver genes at a gland-by-gland level (A) within a human adenoma containing a focus of invasion revealed spatially variegated clones and no clonal sweeps (B). The lack of clonal sweeps is further illustrated by the inferred phylogenetic tree (C). With permission from Thirlwell et al [27].

speed and success of a clone's growth. This stochasticity is an important feature of cancer progression that is not highlighted in the multistep model.

A BIG BANG

Recently, a new model of colorectal cancer growth termed the 'Big Bang' (**Figure 3.3**) has been proposed [49], which is in stark contrast to the sequential model. The Big Bang model is summarised as follows:

- The Big Bang model proposes that colorectal cancers (CRCs) grow as a single (clonal) expansion, rather than evolving sequentially via multiple selective sweeps.
- The Big Bang model proposes the composition of subclones that naturally arise within the single expansion do not experience stringent (differential) selection. This means that subclones do not 'grow out' or, in other words, that acquiring a new driver mutation does not trigger a selective sweep. Therefore, extensive intratumour heterogeneity is expected. A corollary of this is that all clones within a Big Bang tumour must grow at approximately the same rate as one another.
- Because of the lack of selection, it is the timing of a mutation, rather than selection for that mutation, that is the principle determinant of clone size within the tumour. This means that mutations arising early will tend to form large subclones, whereas mutations arising later will form clones of restricted size.

The Big Bang model was postulated to explain the results of a detailed genetic analysis of intratumour diversity in colorectal cancers and adenomas. The spatial distribution of point mutations and copy number alterations across different regions of these tumours was recorded, and a computational modelling approach was used to determine the most likely way in which the tumour would grow. This revealed that a sequential model, whereby each sizeable subclone was generated by the clonal selection of a mutant that occurred late-on in tumour development, was extremely unlikely to explain the observed spatial distribution of subclones. Instead, the computational analysis predicted that all the sizeable subclones arose early during the cancer expansion, and that their size was not strongly determined by their fitness. The conclusion was reached through an explicit consideration of the conspicuous (but ironically often neglected) fact that a tumour consists of an almost

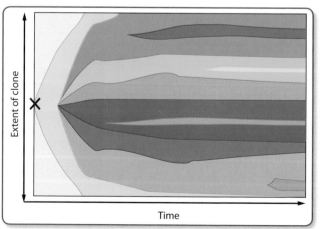

Figure 3.3 Clonal expansions in the Big Bang model of colon cancer growth. The initial events in tumour evolution wholly determine the later clonal composition of the tumour. All sizeable clonal expansions occur early in tumour growth, whereas later occurring clones are unable to grow to an appreciable size. Clonal sweeps do not occur. Adapted from Sottoriva et al [49].

Extent of clone

Time

innumerable population of cells. For example, a 1-cm^3 tumour is considered to be at the lower size limit of clinical detection, but already contains approximately one billion (10^9) cells, which required many millions of cell divisions to grow. This is a prescient feature when thinking about the clonal expansions, because in large and growing populations it is extremely difficult for sizeable clonal expansions to occur. The reasons for this are (1) that to grow to a detectable size within a large population it requires a similarly large clonal expansion, which is likely to take an unfeasibly long time, especially since the expansion of a new clone will be slowed by competition with the resident clone on its periphery [50,51]; (2) sweeps to fixation in a growing population are extremely difficult to achieve, as the growth rate of a new subclone must dramatically exceed the growth rate of the resident population for a sustained period of time. Measurements of the selective advantage of new driver mutations might make it seem physiological possible for a new subclone to evolve a drastically elevated growth rate (for instance, *KRAS* mutants experience a fivefold selective advantage over wild-type cells within the intestinal crypt [52]), but it is important to bear in mind that a selective sweep through a growing tumour requires the new clone to compete with the resident tumour cells that already, themselves, have elevated fitness. In other words, the differential increase in fitness bestowed by a new driver mutation is likely to be much less within a tumour than in the mutant versus wild-type situations that have been analysed to date (indeed, mathematical modelling estimates that the fitness increase bestowed a new driver mutation in human cancers are as low as 1% [53]).

In summary, the computational simulations of subclone evolution in a growing tumour showed that late-arising subclones were extremely unlikely to expand to the sizes detected by multiregion sampling, and rather that observed subclonal topology was readily explained by the accrual of the subclone defining mutations during the initial expansion of the tumour [49]. Importantly, the size of these early-arising subclone mutations was not strongly influenced by the strength of clonal selection they experienced. Consequently, the large population size, and perhaps initial rapid growth rate of colorectal tumours, means that diversity within Big Bang tumours is essentially fixed over time, and that appreciable diversity can only be generated during the initial growth of the tumour when the population size of the tumour is small enough for new clones to become established and sweep through the population. Herein lies the reason for the naming of the Big Bang model: it proposes that the clonal composition of a tumour, at least at a macroscopic level, is determined early on and remains effectively static thereafter; this is analogous to the cosmological model wherein perturbations during the initial expansion of the universe still dominate in the modern day cosmic microwave background [49]. Clinically, the Big Bang model raises the intriguing question of whether cancers are 'born to be bad': if the clonal composition of the tumour is essentially fixed from the outset of tumour growth, it is logical to think that the early events will determine the prognosis of the tumour, and perhaps its sensitivity to treatment. This is clearly an avenue for future research.

It is as yet undetermined whether Big Bang dynamics are observed in other cancer types, but it is our opinion that the causes of Big Bang evolutionary dynamics described above could apply equally well in other tumour types.

PUNCTUATED EQUILIBRIA AND HOPEFUL MONSTERS

The sequential model assumes that driver mutations accrue sequentially, and that each driver bestows a large increase in fitness to the recipient clone. This is an example of phyletic gradualism where phenotypic evolution proceeds in an incremental fashion (a hypothetical example is the steady ramping up of a cell's proliferative rate over time as driver mutations accrue). Clearly, the Big Bang model is at odds with phyletic gradualism: the Big Bang model proposes that the significant selection occurs at the outset of cancer growth (or at least at the time of the last expansion) and that subsequent evolutionary selection within the expanding population is of negligible magnitude and/or consequence. The Big Bang model is thus an example of punctuated equilibrium [54] whereby large phenotypic leaps can suddenly occur in an otherwise phenotypically static population (in the Big Bang model, the phenotypic leap is the switch from no expansion to the initiation of a large rapid expansion).

It is important to note that a punctuated equilibria evolutionary model is a model purely of the pattern of phenotypic change in a population but makes no comment on the pattern of genotypic change. The relationship between genotype and phenotype is complex, because small genotypic changes can have large phenotypic consequences (take the single base-pair changes in the *APC* or other genes that can cause hereditary polyposis syndromes [55] as a good example) and because a cell's phenotype is defined in conjunction with its microenvironment. Nevertheless, it is intriguing to ask whether large changes in genotype underpin the phenotypic leaps. Following Goldschmidt's conjecture, individuals with grossly altered genomes are referred to as 'hopeful monsters', where the 'hopefulness' derives from the chance that the alterations will provide some (significant) increase in fitness to the mutated individual.

Is the development of a hopeful monster a plausible cause of a Big Bang? This is the question we address in the remainder of this review.

GENETIC INSTABILITY, CHROMOSOMAL CATASTROPHES AND CONSPIRING CLONES

Genetic instability has long been recognised as a hallmark of cancer [11]. In the colon, the significant majority of cancers (about 85%) show large-scale chromosomal rearrangements and are labelled as having chromosomal instability (CIN), a phenotype where gross karyotypic alterations, such as the loss and gain of whole chromosome arms, occur at an elevated rate [56]. The remaining 15% of colorectal cancers have elevated point mutation rates that are attributable to defects in mismatch repair [MMR; these defects also cause microsatellite instability (MSI), hence MMR-deficient cancers are usually referred to as MSI+] or defects in other DNA replication and repair enzymes [57]. Both CIN and MIN causes elevated rates of ongoing genetic change, and can clearly increase the rate at which fitness increasing (driver) mutations accrue [58].

A steady accrual of mutations (either at an elevated or at a basal rate) could underpin punctuated evolution if certain conditions about the relationship between genotype and phenotype are met: (1) driver mutations must be rare enough that periods of time sufficient for a selective sweep elapse between each sequential driver mutation and (2) the accrual of a single new driver mutation must cause a significant change in phenotype. A more complete characterisation of the driver mutations in different tumour types is needed [10] before it is possible to determine if these conditions are met.

Intriguingly, recent developments in whole genome sequencing technologies have led to the identification of a new class of mutational processes that cause enormous changes to the genome in a single or very few cell divisions. These include chromothripsis – the shattering of a chromosome into many parts and their (partial) reassembly into a different order [59,60] – and chromoplexy – interleaved chromosomal alterations that involve multiple chromosomes [61]. The clustering of somatic point mutations in localised regions of the genome, a process termed kataegis, has also been observed [62] although how these mutations are accrued over time is unknown [63,64]. While as yet unstudied, an appealing hypothesis is that it is a 'chromosomal catastrophe' of this sort that leads to the generation of a hopeful monster and the subsequent initiation of a Big Bang.

Noncell-autonomous effects, such as the production of a growth factor by one clone and its use by another, can also be drivers of a clonal expansion in tumours [65,66]. This is a pertinent point, as it demonstrates that phenotypic changes need not be elicited by genotypic changes in the expanding clone.

CONCLUSION

What are the practical consequences of these considerations? One important issue is the way in which we look at the early diagnosis of cancer by the identification of premalignant lesions. Let us look at two well-established lesions that are currently the subject of world-wide screening and surveillance programmes – the colorectal adenoma, now universally considered to be the precursor to colorectal cancer, and Barrett's oesophagus.

Conventional colorectal adenomas are known to have a long life history, often sitting in the colon in a state of evolutionary stasis for many years [67] – estimated to be as many as 10–15 years [17] – and progressing through punctuated genetic events to eventually develop the invasive phenotype [49]. Many such lesions do not progress and it is presently not possible to predict which lesions will go on to become invasive. The fact that genetic progression occurs in spatially segregated clones [27] is immaterial – because the whole adenoma is removed. However, once invasion occurs there is a 'flat' clonal expansion [68], and progression to an advanced carcinoma can then be quite rapid. But, within the context of a screening programme, because there is a wide window in which intervention can remove the whole lesion, being able to anticipate and thus prevent the invasive event is critical. Of course, for patients with resected adenomas, there is then the question of what will happen in the future to the patient, and indeed whether it is possible, by looking at the genotype/phenotype of the index adenoma(s) to predict future cancer risk. In the context of the Big Bang model described above, the question is whether or not an imminent Big Bang can be detected before the 'explosion' happens. This is the subject of current research.

But consider the case of Barrett's oesophagus: here too, most Barrett's segments exist in a state of evolutionary stasis – so-called nonprogressors. However, in patients who do progress (progressors) to dysplasia and carcinoma, the situation is quite different. It is now clear (as we have seen above) that genetic progression in Barrett's oesophagus does not progress in selective sweeps involving the whole Barrett's segment, but occurs through individual clones that expand independently [69] and often this can be a very focal event [25,26]. Barrett's segments can be long – over 10 cm, and even the most invasive screening/surveillance protocols cannot be expected to pick up such localised events. Moreover, it is now clear that progression to carcinoma can be fairly rapid, with the apparently critical somatic copy-number alterations occurring within a 3–4-year window [25,26]. Progression to cancer in Barrett's oesophagus is both localised and rapid; this puts considerable constraints on the design of effective screening/surveillance programmes. On the other hand, there is evidence to suggest that it is possible to stratify patients at risk of progression at an early stage from the genetic diversity across the Barrett's segment [70], or from the complement of mutant clones present [71,72].

It is often said that models of the genetic progression to cancer have limited translational potential. We propose that finding the right model for cancer progression could be rate limiting for the design of appropriate methods of preventing and treating cancer.

Key points for clinical practice

- Most pre-malignant and pre-invasive lesions, such as DCIS, colorectal adenomas and Barrett's oesophagus are in a state of evolutionary stasis – most will not progress to malignancy.

- In a number of tumour types the main driver mutations occur early in the neoplastic process: thus the behaviour of the tumour will be fixed at the outset – `born to be bad'.

- The rate of evolutionary tumour progression can be very fast, and may be the basis of `interval cancers', missed on surveillance in, for example, Barrett's oesophagus.

- It has to be the focus of future research to identify those pre-malignant and pre-invasive lesions which are destined to progress, and to predict those cancers where progression is likely to be rapid and to tailor therapy appropriately.

REFERENCES

1.   Wright NA. Boveri at 100: cancer evolution, from preneoplasia to malignancy. J Pathol 2014; 234:146–151.
2.   Tyzzer E. Tumor immunity. J Cancer Res 1916; 1:125–126.
3.   Armitage P, Doll R. The age distribution of cancer and a multi-stage theory of carcinogenesis. Br J Cancer 1954; 8:1–12.
4.   Knudson AG. Mutation and cancer: statistical study of retinoblastoma. Proc Natl Acad Sci USA 1971; 68:820–823.
5.   Fearon ER, Vogelstein B. A genetic model for colorectal tumorigenesis. Cell 1990; 61:759–767.
6.   Kinzler KW, Vogelstein B. Lessons from hereditary colorectal cancer. Cell 1996; 87:159–170.
7.   Hruban RH, Goggins M, Parsons J, et al. Progression model for pancreatic cancer. Clin Cancer Res 2000; 6:2969–2972.
8.   Polyak K. On the birth of breast cancer. Biochim Biophys Acta 2001; 1552:1–13.
9.   Nowell PC. The clonal evolution of tumor cell populations. Science 1976; 194:23–28.
10.   Greaves M. Evolutionary determinants of cancer. Cancer Discov 2015; 5:806–820.
11.   Hanahan D, Weinberg RA. The hallmarks of cancer. Cell 2000;100:57–70.
12.   Hanahan D, Weinberg RA. Hallmarks of cancer: the next generation. Cell 2011;144:646–674.
13.   Visvader JE. Cells of origin in cancer. Nature 2011; 469:314–322.
14.   Maley CC, Galipeau PC, Li X, et al. Selectively advantageous mutations and hitchhikers in neoplasms: p16 lesions are selected in Barrett's esophagus. Cancer Res 2004; 64:3414–3427.
15.   Maley CC, Reid BJ. Natural selection in neoplastic progression of Barrett's esophagus. Semin Cancer Biol 2005; 15:474–483.
16.   McDonald SA, Lavery D, Wright NA, et al. Barrett oesophagus: lessons on its origins from the lesion itself. Nat Rev Gastroenterol Hepatol 2015; 12:50–60.
17.   Jones S, Chen WD, Parmigiani G, et al. Comparative lesion sequencing provides insights into tumor evolution. Proc Natl Acad Sci U S A 2008; 105:4283–4288.
18.   Sprouffske K, Pepper JW, Maley CC. Accurate reconstruction of the temporal order of mutations in neoplastic progression. Cancer Prev Res (Phila) 2011; 4:1135–1144.
19.   Barker N, Ridgway RA, van Es JH, et al. Crypt stem cells as the cells-of-origin of intestinal cancer. Nature 2009; 457:608–611.
20.   Clevers H. The cancer stem cell: premises, promises and challenges. Nature Med 2011; 17:313–319.
21.   Salk JJ, Fox EJ, Loeb LA. Mutational heterogeneity in human cancers: origin and consequences. Ann Rev Pathol 2010; 5:51–75.
22.   Sieber OM, Tomlinson SR, Tomlinson IPM. Tissue, cell and stage specificity of (epi)mutations in cancers. Nature Rev Cancer 2005; 5:649–655.

23. Martincorena I, Roshan A, Gerstung M, et al. Tumor evolution. High burden and pervasive positive selection of somatic mutations in normal human skin. Science 2015; 348:880–886.
24. Galandiuk S, Rodriguez-Justo M, Jeffery R, et al. Field cancerization in the intestinal epithelium of patients with Crohn's ileocolitis. Gastroenterology 2012; 142:855–864.e8.
25. Kostadinov RL, Kuhner MK, Li X, et al. NSAIDs modulate clonal evolution in Barrett's esophagus. PLoS Genet 2013; 9:e1003553.
26. Li X, Galipeau PC, Paulson TG, et al. Temporal and spatial evolution of somatic chromosomal alterations: a case-cohort study of Barrett's esophagus. Cancer Prev Res (Phila) 2014; 7:114–127.
27. Thirlwell C, Will OC, Domingo E, et al. Clonality assessment and clonal ordering of individual neoplastic crypts shows polyclonality of colorectal adenomas. Gastroenterology 2010; 138:1441–1454, 1454.e1-1454.e7.
28. Humphries A, Cereser B, Gay LJ, et al. Lineage tracing reveals multipotent stem cells maintain human adenomas and the pattern of clonal expansion in tumor evolution. Proc Natl Acad Sci U S A 2013; 110: E2490–E2499.
29. Marusyk A, Almendro V, Polyak K. Intra-tumour heterogeneity: a looking glass for cancer? Nat Rev Cancer 2012; 12:323–334.
30. Gerlinger M, Rowan AJ, Horswell S, et al. Intratumor heterogeneity and branched evolution revealed by multiregion sequencing. N Engl J Med 2012; 366:883–892.
31. Gerlinger M, Horswell S, Larkin J, et al. Genomic architecture and evolution of clear cell renal cell carcinomas defined by multiregion sequencing. Nat Genet 2014; 46:225–233.
32. de Bruin EC, McGranahan N, Mitter R, et al. Spatial and temporal diversity in genomic instability processes defines lung cancer evolution. Science 2014; 346:251–256.
33. Zhang J, Fujimoto J, Zhang J, et al. Intratumor heterogeneity in localized lung adenocarcinomas delineated by multiregion sequencing. Science 2014; 346:256–259.
34. Shah SP, Roth A, Goya R, et al. The clonal and mutational evolution spectrum of primary triple-negative breast cancers. Nature 2012; 486:395–399.
35. Nik-Zainal S, Van Loo P, Wedge DC, et al. The life history of 21 breast cancers. Cell 2012; 149:994–1007.
36. Yates LR, Gerstung M, Knappskog S, et al. Subclonal diversification of primary breast cancer revealed by multiregion sequencing. Nat Med 2015; 21:751–759.
37. Sottoriva A, Spiteri I, Piccirillo SG, et al. Intratumor heterogeneity in human glioblastoma reflects cancer evolutionary dynamics. Proc Natl Acad Sci USA 2013; 110:4009–4014.
38. Johnson BE, Mazor T, Hong C, et al. Mutational analysis reveals the origin and therapy-driven evolution of recurrent glioma. Science 2014; 343:189–193.
39. Anderson K, Lutz C, van Delft FW, et al. Genetic variegation of clonal architecture and propagating cells in leukaemia. Nature 2011; 469: 356–361.
40. Schwarz RF, Ng CK, Cooke SL, et al. Spatial and temporal heterogeneity in high-grade serous ovarian cancer: a phylogenetic analysis. PLoS Med 2015; 12:e1001789.
41. Okosun J, Bödör C, Wang J, et al. Integrated genomic analysis identifies recurrent mutations and evolution patterns driving the initiation and progression of follicular lymphoma. Nat Genet 2014; 46:176–181.
42. Ding L, Ley TJ, Larson DE, et al. Clonal evolution in relapsed acute myeloid leukaemia revealed by whole-genome sequencing. Nature 2012; 481: 506–510.
43. Yachida S, Jones S, Bozic I, et al. Distant metastasis occurs late during the genetic evolution of pancreatic cancer. Nature 2010; 467: 1114–1117.
44. Gundem G, Van Loo P, Kremeyer B, et al. The evolutionary history of lethal metastatic prostate cancer. Nature 2015; 520: 353–357.
45. Driessens G, Beck B, Caauwe A, et al. Defining the mode of tumour growth by clonal analysis. Nature 2012; 488:527–530.
46. Vermeulen L, Morrissey E, van der Heijden M, et al. Defining stem cell dynamics in models of intestinal tumor initiation. Science 2013; 342: 995–998.
47. Baker AM, Cereser B, Melton S, et al. Quantification of crypt and stem cell evolution in the normal and neoplastic human colon. Cell Rep 2014; 8: 940–947.
48. Teixeira VH, Nadarajan P, Graham TA, et al. Stochastic homeostasis in human airway epithelium is achieved by neutral competition of basal cell progenitors. Elife 2013; 2:e00966.
49. Sottoriva A, Kang H, Ma Z, et al. A Big Bang model of human colorectal tumor growth. Nat Genet 2015; 47:209–216.
50. Chao DL, Eck JT, Brash DE, et al. Preneoplastic lesion growth driven by the death of adjacent normal stem cells. Proc Natl Acad Sci USA 2008; 105:15034–15039.

51. Martens EA, Kostadinov R, Maley CC, et al. Spatial structure increases the waiting time for cancer. New J Phys 2011; 13:115014.
52. Snippert HJ, Schepers AG, van Es JH, et al. Biased competition between Lgr5 intestinal stem cells driven by oncogenic mutation induces clonal expansion. EMBO Rep 2014; 15:62–69.
53. Bozic I, Antal T, Ohtsuki H, et al. Accumulation of driver and passenger mutations during tumor progression. Proc Natl Acad Sci USA 2010; 107:18545–18550.
54. Eldredge N, Jay GS. Punctuated equilibria: an alternative to phyletic gradualism. In: Schopf TJM (ed.), Models in paleobiology. San Francisco: Freeman, Cooper, 1972:82–115.
55. Tomlinson I. An update on the molecular pathology of the intestinal polyposis syndromes. Diagn Histopathol 2015; 21:147–151.
56. Lengauer C, Kinzler KW, Vogelstein B. Genetic instability in colorectal cancers. Nature 1997; 386:623–627.
57. Cancer Genome Atlas Network. Comprehensive molecular characterization of human colon and rectal cancer. Nature 2012; 487:330–337.
58. Loeb LA. Human cancers express mutator phenotypes: origin, consequences and targeting. Nat Rev Cancer 2011; 11:450–457.
59. Stephens PJ, Greenman CD, Fu B, et al. Massive genomic rearrangement acquired in a single catastrophic event during cancer development. Cell 2011; 144: 27–40.
60. Zhang CZ, Spektor A, Cornils H, et al. Chromothripsis from DNA damage in micronuclei. Nature 2015; 522:179–184.
61. Baca SC, Prandi D, Lawrence MS, et al. Punctuated evolution of prostate cancer genomes. Cell 2013; 153:666–677.
62. Nik-Zainal S, Alexandrov LB, Wedge DC, et al. Mutational processes molding the genomes of 21 breast cancers. Cell 2012; 149: 979–993.
63. Sakofsky CJ, Roberts SA, Malc E, et al. Break-induced replication is a source of mutation clusters underlying kataegis. Cell Rep 2014; 7:1640–1648.
64. Fischer A, Illingworth CJ, Campbell PJ, et al. EMu: probabilistic inference of mutational processes and their localization in the cancer genome. Genome Biol 2013; 14:R39.
65. Marusyk A, Tabassum DP, Altrock PM, et al. Non-cell-autonomous driving of tumour growth supports sub-clonal heterogeneity. Nature 2014; 514:54–58.
66. Cleary AS, Leonard TL, Gestl SA, et al. Tumour cell heterogeneity maintained by cooperating subclones in Wnt-driven mammary cancers. Nature 2014; 508:113–117.
67. Hofstad B, Vatn MH, Andersen SN, et al. Growth of colorectal polyps: redetection and evaluation of unresected polyps for a period of three years. Gut 1996; 39:449–456.
68. Siegmund K, Marjoram P, Woo YJ, et al. Inferring clonal expansion and cancer stem cell dynamics from DNA methylation patterns in colorectal cancers. Proc Natl Acad Sci USA 2009; 106:4828–4833.
69. Leedham SJ, Preston SL, McDonald SA, et al. Individual crypt genetic heterogeneity and the origin of metaplastic glandular epithelium in human Barrett's oesophagus. Gut 2008; 57:1041–1048.
70. Maley CC, Galipeau PC, Finley JC, et al. Genetic clonal diversity predicts progression to esophageal adenocarcinoma. Nature Genet 2006; 38: 468–473.
71. Maley CC, Galipeau PC, Li X, et al. The combination of genetic instability and clonal expansion predicts progression to esophageal adenocarcinoma. Cancer Res 2004; 64:7629–7633.
72. Timmer MR, Martinez P, Lau CT, et al. Derivation of genetic biomarkers for cancer risk stratification in Barrett's oesophagus: a prospective cohort study. Gut 2015; pii: gutjnl-2015-309642.

Chapter 4

Molecular profiling of osteoarticular neoplasms

Adrienne M Flanagan, Fernanda Amary

INTRODUCTION

Data generated from large-scale sequencing of DNA and RNA from bone tumours has revealed highly recurrent alterations which for the most part are mutually exclusive for the different tumour types. This has transformed the ability of pathologists to distinguish tumours with overlapping histological features. These findings are already being exploited and have been introduced as part of the laboratory diagnostic armoury. The next phase of research in this area will be to determine if genetic profiles of bone tumours can be employed as prognostic and predictive markers and if targeted therapies can be developed against these alterations.

CARTILAGINOUS TUMOURS

Benign and malignant cartilaginous tumours represent the most common group of primary bone tumour. By far, the most common subtypes are benign conventional cartilaginous tumours – osteochondromas sited on the bone surface and enchondromas sited centrally within the medullary space. Both may transform into chondrosarcoma. Close to 85% of conventional chondrosarcomas are sited centrally, and the remaining, 10–15% occur on the bone surface. There is also a rare surface variant, the periosteal chondroma, but it is exceptional for this tumour to progress to chondrosarcoma.

It has been known for some time that osteochondromas are characterised by the presence of *EXT1* and *EXT2* mutations [1].

IDH1 and *IDH2* in central conventional and dedifferentiated cartilaginous tumours

In 2011, we reported that approximately 60% of conventional central and periosteal cartilaginous tumours harbour a mutation in *IDH1* or *IDH2* with the majority occurring in *IDH1,* and only approximately 6% in *IDH2* R172 but not in R140 which is usually

Adrienne M Flanagan MD PhD FRCPath FMedSci, University College London Cancer Institute, London and the Royal National Orthopaedic Hospital NHS Trust, Stanmore, UK. Email: a.flanagan@ucl.ac.uk (for correspondence)

Fernanda Amary MD PhD, Royal National Orthopaedic Hospital NHS Trust, Stanmore, UK

found in myeloid neoplasms (**Table 4.1, Figure 4.1**). These mutations are never seen in osteochondromas, peripheral chondrosarcomas (secondary to osteochondromas) or synovial chondromatosis [2,3]. The same mutations are seen in glioblastomas, in a proportion of acute myeloid leukaemia, and cholangiocarcinomas and other tumours much less commonly. Of note is that the incidence of the specific mutations in the different tumours varies. The *IDH1/IDH2* mutations are present in all grades of central conventional chondrosarcoma, and in dedifferentiated chondrosarcoma. If present, they are always detected at the time of the presentation of the disease, and persist throughout its course, being found in both local recurrences and metastatic lesions [4].

The mutant IDH1/IDH2 enzyme fails to convert isocitrate to α-ketoglutarate, and gains a new function that leads to the accumulation of D-2-hydroxyglutarate (2HG) which provides the properties of an oncometabolite and tumour-inducing actions. Just as reported for *IDH1/IDH2* mutation-harbouring brain tumours, we demonstrated high levels of 2HG in cartilaginous tumours with these mutations, and demonstrated that they were hypermethylated [5].

Table 4.1 Genetic abnormalities underlying bone tumours	
Aneurysmal bone cyst	*USP6* gene rearrangement
Conventional central chondrosarcoma, high grade	*IDH1* or *IDH2* mutation and other alterations including *CDKN2A*
Nonconventional dedifferentiated central chondrosarcoma	*IDH1* or *IDH2* mutation and other alterations
Conventional central chondrosarcoma, low grade/enchondromas	*IDH1* or *IDH2* mutation
Chondroblastoma	*H3F3B* (p.K36M) mutation
Chondromyxoid fibroma	Complex *GRM1* gene rearrangement
Chordoma	*T* (*brachyury*) copy-number gain
Epithelioid hemangioendothelioma	*WWTR1-CAMTA1*
Ewing sarcoma[†]	*EWSR1-FLI1*
	EWSR1-ERG
	FUS-ERG
Ewing-like tumours	*BCOR-CCNB3*
	CIC-DUX4[*]
Fibrous dysplasia	*GNAS1* substitution
Giant cell tumour of bone	*H3F3A* (p.G34W, rarely G34L/M/R) substitution
Mesenchymal chondrosarcoma	*HEY1-NCOA2*
Osteosarcoma, central high grade	*FGFR1* gene amplification
Parosteal and low grade central osteosarcoma	*MDM2* gene amplification
Peripheral chondrosarcoma/osteochondroma	*EXT1* or *EXT2* mutation
Pseudomyogenic haemangioendothelioma	*SERPINE1-FOSB*

[*]Soft tissue tumour.
[†]See Table 4.2 for rare variants involving *EWSR1*.

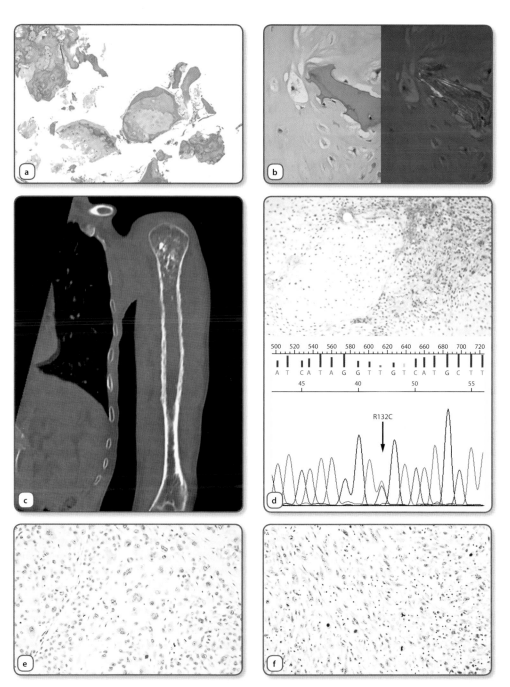

Figure 4.1 Central conventional cartilaginous tumours. (a) Enchondroma showing abundant matrix and tumour nodules encased by a rim of bone. (b) Chondrosarcoma grade I with mature lamellar host bone (emphasised under birefringent light microscopy) which is scalloped on all aspects and entrapped within the tumour. (c) Magnetic resonance imaging of a high-grade chondrosarcoma showing an extensive intramedullary tumour with cortical irregularities. (d) Chondrosarcoma grade II showing cell spindling and nuclei with an open chromatin pattern. Sequencing revealed an IDH1 p.R132C alteration. (e) Chondrosarcoma grade III featuring severe cytological atypia. (f) Dedifferentiated chondrosarcoma featuring a high-grade spindle cell sarcoma component, not otherwise specified.

In addition to *IDH1/IDH2* alterations in chondrosarcoma, exome and whole genome sequencing revealed that *TP53* and *CDKN2A* are common alterations in high-grade chondrosarcomas, occurring in both central and surface variants. Furthermore, 40% of chondrosarcoma harbours a genetic alteration involving *COL2A1*, and 27%, and 22% carry alterations in genes involving the *RB1* and hedgehog signalling pathway respectively, the latter include *SUFU, GLI, PTCH, TULP3, RUNX2, PRRX1* and *HHIP* [6].

Diagnostic value of IDH1/IDH2 mutations

The detection of an *IDH1/IDH2* mutation is particularly helpful in distinguishing dedifferentiated chondrosarcoma containing an osteosarcomatous component from a primary osteosarcoma of bone. This has important therapeutic implications, as osteosarcomas are generally treated with neoadjuvant chemotherapy, whereas this is not the case for chondrosarcomas.

The *IDH1* mutations in chondrosarcoma are also mutually exclusive with the protein expression of brachyury [2], the diagnostic hallmark of chordoma, and with the *HEY1-NCOA2* fusion transcript characteristic of mesenchymal chondrosarcoma (vide infra).

Multiple enchondromas

The clinical entity known as multiple enchondromas represents a genetically disparate group of diseases with a spectrum of overlapping phenotypes [7]. By far the most common variant is Ollier disease, followed by Maffucci syndrome; the latter is characterised by multiple enchondroma-associated soft tissue haemangiomas; both are nonfamilial disorders. Affected individuals are also at risk of developing other noncartilaginous cancers the most common of which is glioblastoma. An *IDH1* or an *IDH2* mutation occurs in the tumours of >90% of individual affected by these allelic disorders, and each tumour in an affected individual carries the same genetic alteration, thereby demonstrating that Ollier disease and Maffucci syndrome represent mosaic disorders [8,9].

Rarer variants of multiple enchondroma include metachondromatosis and spondyloenchondrodysplasia; some of these have recently been linked to specific germline alterations, including *PTPN11*, which encodes protein tyrosine phosphatase, nonreceptor type 11 and *ACP5*, which encodes tartrate-resistant acid phosphatase. *PTHR1* alterations are also associated with a form of multiple enchondromas [2], and others remain to be identified. As these disease entities have overlapping phenotypes, recognition of these mutations will allow robust disease classification that can be employed for diagnosis and stratification for treatment.

Potential new therapeutic options

The mutations in the *IDH1/IDH2* genes were identified in 2008 in brain tumours [10] but already inhibitors are being tested in clinical trials. In addition, a vaccine targeting mutant IDH1 has been developed and shows promising results in mice [11]. The speed at which these therapeutic agents are being developed is remarkable and is a sign of how the genetic classification of disease is driving novel focussed approaches to treating cancer [12].

Mesenchymal chondrosarcoma

This is a nonconventional chondrosarcoma representing only 2% of all chondrosarcomas. Although more commonly occurring in bone, it also presents in soft tissue. This tumour is more frequently sited in the vertebral bodies and in the head and neck region, but can occur anywhere in the body. The highest incidence is within the second and third decades.

The histological features of a mesenchymal chondrosarcoma comprise a biphasic pattern composed of a densely cellular population of primitive neoplastic cells, often arranged in a haemangiopericytic pattern. These tumour cells are strongly immunoreactive for CD99 and can be mistaken for Ewing sarcoma. This cellular component alternates abruptly with an osseous cartilaginous matrix-rich component. In areas the cartilaginous material can be hyaline in nature and can be interpreted as a low-grade conventional chondrosarcoma, whereas if the matrix reveals a more osseous appearance, the differential diagnosis includes osteosarcoma.

In 2003, Marc Ladanyi and his team identified a novel recurrent fusion transcript involving *HEY1-NCOA2* using exon expression data followed by rapid amplification of cDNA ends (RACE) polymerase chain reaction (PCR) [13]. This fusion transcript appears to be specific for the tumour type, and interphase fluorescence in situ hybridisation (FISH) using either dual coloured probes covering both genes (fusion assay) or reverse transcription polymerase chain reaction (RT-PCR) can now be employed in the clinical setting for diagnostic purposes.

The value of chemo- and radiotherapy in the treatment of mesenchymal chondrosarcoma is unclear. The benefit of diagnosing mesenchymal chondrosarcoma on the basis of the *HEY1-NCOA2* fusion means that consistent and reliable diagnoses can be provided, and incorrect diagnoses of Ewing sarcoma, osteosarcoma and conventional chondrosarcoma can be avoided.

Chondromyxoid fibroma

This is a benign primary nonconventional cartilaginous tumour. The peak incidence occurs in the second and third decades. Surgery is the standard treatment and the prognosis is excellent: local recurrence is not infrequent but can be managed conservatively. Histologically, chondromyxoid fibroma shows a multilobulated pattern comprising spindle-shaped and stellate cells embedded in a myxoid matrix and intersected by septa of osteoclast-rich fibrous tissue. Marker nuclear pleomorphism may occur and can be misinterpreted resulting in a misdiagnosis of a malignant tumour (**Figure 4.2**).

Nord et al have recently identified that structural rearrangements involving promoter swapping and gene fusion events result in aberrant expression of the glutamate receptor gene, *GRM1*. This represents a highly specific driver event in the development of this disease [14]. *GRM1* is one of eight metabotropic glutamate receptors denoted *GRM1-GRM8*, all of which are G protein-coupled receptors (**Figure 4.3**).

OSTEOCLAST-RICH NEOPLASMS

The differential diagnosis of an osteoclast-rich neoplasm in bone is wide and includes reactive lesions (to trauma, infection and metabolic disturbances), germline disorders, and benign and highly malignant neoplasms. Making the correct diagnosis on the biopsy is critical as this determines the appropriate clinical treatment. In the case of benign tumours, the treatment is generally curettage with or without local adjuvant agents to the curetted area. In contrast, for high-grade malignant disease the treatment potentially involves neoadjuvant chemotherapy followed by surgical resection with a wide margin.

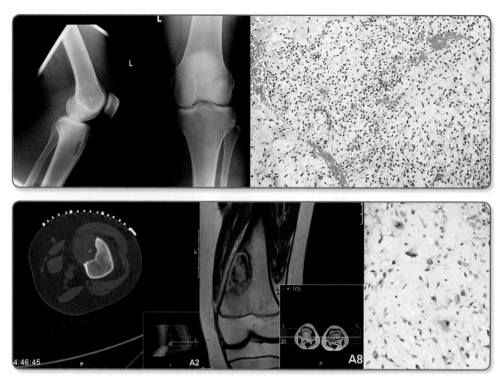

Figure 4.2 Two cases of chondromyxoid fibroma. Upper row: an eccentric lytic lesion in the metaphysis of the proximal tibia. Histological features include bland spindle–stellate cells in a myxoid background. Lower row: an eccentric metaphyseal lesion in the distal femur with well-defined sclerotic margins seen on magnetic resonance imaging and a computerised tomography scan. Photomicrograph shows moderate nuclear atypia which can lead to a misdiagnosis of malignancy.

In the recent past, the genetic alterations of a number of osteoclast-rich lesions have been described and these are now employed to provide more robust diagnoses in the clinical setting. Specifically, *USP6* fusion transcripts occur in approximately 70% of aneurysmal bone cysts (ABCs; vide infra) [15], and whole genomic analysis using massively parallel DNA sequencing revealed a recurrent mutation in either the *H3F3A* or the *H3F3B* gene in six chondroblastomas and in the *H3F3A* gene in five giant cell tumours (GCTs) of bone. The mutations were detected in the stromal cell component and not in the osteoclasts or their precursors [16]. The genomes of both tumour types had low mutational burdens with neither significant copy number nor structural aberrations, specifically *TP53* and *IDH1/IDH2* mutations. *H3F3A* and *H3F3B* encode the replication-independent histone variants H3.3; they occur on chromosomes 1 and 17, respectively, and have different exonic and intronic DNA sequences but they share identical protein sequences. Notably, H3.3 genetic alterations were previously reported in aggressive brain tumours which also harbour *TP53* alterations. H3.3 mutations are mutually exclusive with *USP6* alterations [17].

Giant cell tumour of bone

This is virtually always present in the subarticular (epiphyseal) site of the mature skeleton. The most common sites are the distal femur and proximal tibia but GCT can occur in

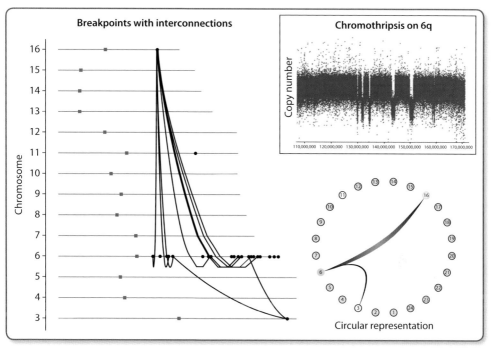

Figure 4.3 Chromothripsis causes complex rearrangement which, at the DNA level, results in a fusion connecting the promoter of *BCLAF1* to *SHPRH* which is sited 5′ to GRM1. At the RNA level this is presumably spliced into the *BCLAF1-GRM1* fusion. By courtesy of Dr Sam Behjati, London, UK.

almost any bone. The histological appearance of a GCT can be varied and includes areas dominated by large osteoclasts, whereas other areas maybe composed of mitotically active spindle cells. Ischaemic necrosis is a frequent occurrence in these tumours.

An *H3F3A* genetic alteration has been detected in >95% of GCT when excluding osteoclast-rich lesions of the bones of hand and feet [16]. An extended study showed that 83/89 of the *H3F3A* alterations involved p.Gly34Trp (p.G34W) and one tumour harboured a p.G34R and one a p.G34M alteration, both of which revealed typical histological appearances and behaved in a nonaggressive fashion. *H3F3B* alterations have never been detected in GCT [16].

GCTs occasionally metastasise to the lungs but such tumours retain the histological features of the primary tumour; the disease can be generally controlled by resection and does not transform into high-grade disease. In the two cases of metastatic GCT to the lung which we studied, the p.G34W alteration was detected in both the primary and metastatic disease and *TP53* alterations were not detected in these lesions.

Others have reported *IDH2* alterations in GCT but we have not been able to confirm these findings in >90 GCT [18].

Chondroblastoma

This is a nonconventional central benign central cartilaginous tumour of bone and share many similarities with GCT of bone; it is sited in the subarticular space and may contain large numbers of osteoclasts, but unlike GCT it can present in the immature skeleton.

Chondroblastoma has a variable and heterogeneous appearance; the cartilaginous component, which is the histological hallmark, may represent a dominant or a small part of the tumour (**Figure 4.4**). More than 95% of chondroblastomas harbour a mutation in either the *H3F3A* or the *H3F3B* genes; these always involve p.Lys36Met (p.K36M). These were mutually exclusive with the *H3F3A* p.G43 W and L mutations in GCT [16,17]. This mutation has not been identified to date in a malignant bone tumour.

Aneurysmal bone cyst

This benign tumour primarily arises in bone but occasionally in soft tissue. It occurs more commonly in children and young adults but has been reported up to the age of 60. The characteristic features are of multiple cysts lined by slim spindle cells, the walls of which are commonly composed of a layer of osteoid along which numerous osteoclasts reside and may protrude into the blood-filled cystic spaces. However, the range of histological features is wide and much of the tumour may be solid, and bone deposition can occur. The neoplastic cells, represented by stromal fibroblast-like cells rather than osteaclasts, may be mitotically active although these are normal in configuration. Necrosis is generally not a feature. It is usually possible to provide the diagnosis on a needle-core biopsy; the differential diagnosis includes other osteoclast-rich lesions

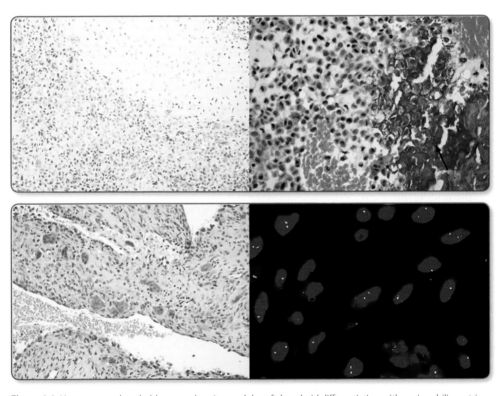

Figure 4.4 Upper row: a chondroblastoma showing nodules of chondroid differentiation with eosinophilic matrix and pericellular chicken-wire calcification (arrow). Lower row: an aneurysmal bone cyst showing blood-filled spaces transected by osteoclast-rich fibrous septa surrounding blood-filled spaces and FISH showing a *USP6* gene rearrangement (break-apart probes).

such as GCT, chondroblastoma and telangiectatic osteosarcoma. The report by Oliveira et al in 2004 showing that close to 70% of ABC contains a *USP6* fusion transcript involving multiple different partners has facilitated the diagnosis of this tumour [15]. Dual-coloured break-apart probes are available commercially and can be used in the diagnostic setting to provide a rapid and robust diagnosis (**Figure 4.4b**). It is notable that *USP6* is also recurrently altered in nodular fasciitis, a soft tissue lesion which has always considered to be a reactive process following trauma. The genetic alteration in this lesion ignites the question of how a neoplasm should be defined [19]. ABC and nodular fasciitis are not dissimilar histologically, with osteoclast-like cells also occurring – although in small numbers – in nodular fasciitis.

Giant cell granuloma of the jaw, and bone of hands and feet

Giant cell lesions of the small bones of the hand and feet and giant cell granuloma of the jaw are distinct entities according to the World Health Organization (WHO) classification [20]. However, it has been considered for some time that at least a proportion of such lesions in the bones of the hand and feet represent a 'solid variant' of ABC, and that true GCT may also occur at these sites. Agaram et al provided evidence for this concept by demonstrating that the eight of nine osteoclast-rich lesions in the small bones of the hands and feet harboured the *USP6* rearrangement characteristic of ABC [21]. Furthermore, they reported that neither eight GCTs (two in the finger) nor eight giant cell granulomas of the jaw harboured a *USP6* alteration. We add weight to this study by showing that of 24 GCTs of the small bones of the hand ($n = 11$) and feet ($n = 13$) studied, 15 harboured an *H3F3A* mutation, 13 of which involved a p.G34W alteration and the other 2 alterations were represented by p.G34L. *USP6* alterations were detected in three of these tumours, all of which were mutually exclusive with the p.G34 alterations. These findings when taken with those of Agram et al argue that tumours classified as GCTs of the small bones of the hand and feet according to the WHO classification (2013) would be better classified as ABC and GCT on the basis of genetic findings [17,20].

Analysis of 78 solitary giant cell granulomas of the jaw did not harbour an *H3F3A* or *H3F3B* alternation [17,22], a finding supported by others [21].

The finding that giant cell granuloma of the jaw and that a small number of GCTs of the small bones of the hand and feet do not exhibit either *USP6* or *H3F3* alterations demonstrates that genetic alteration(s) remain to be identified in these tumours.

Sensitivity and specificity of H3F3A and H3F3B mutations

H3.3 mutations have rarely been reported in malignant bone tumours: they have been reported in 3/110 osteosarcomas (2 involving p.G34R and 1 involving p.G34W), one clear cell chondrosarcoma, 1/75 conventional chondrosarcoma and 1 unusual subarticular tumour with the radiology supporting a diagnosis of a GCT. This last case exhibited a triphasic tumour comprising features of a conventional adamantinoma, alongside a high-grade spindle cell sarcoma part of which contains numerous osteoclasts. Even though this represents a very small number of malignant bone tumours with H3.3 alterations, it means that detection of an H3.3 mutation in an osteoclast-rich tumour cannot exclude a diagnosis of malignancy. Nevertheless, as at least 95% of GCT and chondroblastoma harbour an H3.3 mutation, these diagnoses should be made with caution in the absence of the relevant H3.3 alteration [17].

BONE-FORMING NEOPLASMS

High-grade osteosarcoma

This is the most common primary malignant bone tumour, accounting for <1% of all cancers. Since the late 1970s these tumours have been treated with neoadjuvant chemotherapy resulting in a 5-year survival rate of approximately 60% in those patients whose tumours present without metastatic disease, and arise in the appendicular skeleton [20]. However, despite numerous studies involving gene expression and array CGH, it is still not possible to predict which patients with osteosarcoma will benefit from such neoadjuvant chemotherapy. Amplification of fibroblastic growth receptor (*FGFR*) 1 has recently been shown to occur in approximately 20% of all high-grade osteosarcomas; this was only found in cases which failed to respond to chemotherapy [23]. Since inhibitors to *FGFR* signalling are available, this finding provides an opportunity for stratifying patients with this disease and inclusion in clinical trials.

Parosteal and low-grade central osteosarcomas, and fibrous dysplasia

These are bone-forming neoplasms. Histologically, they share many features including irregularly spaced and shaped woven bone trabeculae embedded within a bland spindle cell population of cells in which there is an absence of necrosis and minimal mitotic activity. Distinguishing these three entities is generally achieved by assessment of the imaging; the parosteal osteosarcoma being 'stuck' to the bone surface (**Figure 4.5**), whereas fibrous dysplasia and low-grade central osteosarcoma are centrally based. Nevertheless, a small number of fibrous dysplasia cases are sited eccentrically and protrude onto the surface, giving the name fibrous dysplasia protuberans. Low-grade central osteosarcomas cannot easily be separated from fibrous dysplasia on the basis of imaging as both are centrally placed.

Fibrous dysplasia is a mosaic disorder brought about by a substitution in *GNAS1*, frequently involving codon 201: p.R201H or p.R201C. A small number of genetic alternations occur in codon 227, resulting in p.Q227L [24]. The majority of patients affected by this disorder have a single lesion, but a polyostotic variant occurs which more frequently presents in children. Intramuscular myxoma forms part of the mosaic disorder in which case the syndrome is referred to as Mazabraud syndrome.

Parosteal osteosarcomas and low-grade central osteosarcomas are characterised by *MDM2* gene amplification. This genetic alteration is found in 80–90% of the former and 30% of the latter [20]. In view of the similarities between parosteal osteosarcoma and fibrous dysplasia and the lack of published data on the specificity of the two molecular markers, namely *MDM2* amplification and *GNAS1* substitutions, Carter et al recently assessed nine parosteal osteosarcomas for *GNAS1* amplification [25]. Somewhat surprisingly, they identified that five of nine such tumours harboured a *GNAS1* mutation. In view of this report we screened 55 parosteal osteosarcomas, 27 of which harboured *MDM2* amplification (9 diploid and 19 noninformative), and failed to detect any *GNAS1* mutations; the analysis was undertaken using a variety of highly sensitive technologies including the FLUIDIGM access array system, with subsequent sequencing on the Ion torrent personal genome machine (PGM), in addition to bidirectional capillary sequencing. Any case where an inconclusive result was obtained the DNA was analysed using mutation-specific restriction enzyme digestion as previously reported [26]. Furthermore, to ensure the quality of the DNA was sufficiently high for detection of mutations, digital droplet PCR analysis of the DNA of all cases was undertaken [26].

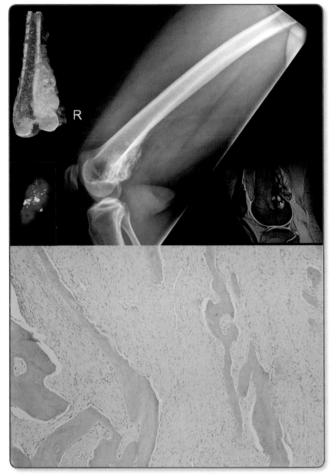

Figure 4.5 A parosteal osteosarcoma illustrated by a plain radiograph showing a calcified mass at the back of the knee (distal femur): the MRI shows an intramedullary extension, with the matching gross specimen. The photomicrograph shows parallel trabeculae of woven and lamellar bone: in the intertrabelular spaces there are fascicles of mildly atypical spindle cells. FISH shows clusters of green signals indicating amplification of the MDM2 gene.

On the basis of failing to detect *GNAS1* mutations in the largest cohort of osteosarcomas to date, including 24 central low-grade osteosarcomas, 11 periosteal osteosarcomas and 55 parosteal osteosarcomas, we conclude that such mutations in parosteal osteosarcomas rarely occur [26]. This supports the previous report by Tabareau-Delalande et al where they failed to find such mutations in 12 parosteal osteosarcomas. There is no obvious explanation for the findings published by Carter et al.

TUMOURS OF UNCERTAIN DIFFERENTIATION

Ewing sarcoma

This is a round cell neoplasm composed of a monotonous cell population with little intervening matrix; it occurs in bone and soft tissue although close to 80% occur in the bone in children and young adults whereas the majority of Ewing sarcoma in soft tissue occurs in adults. Previously, Ewing sarcoma included morphologically similar entities and reported as Askin tumour, and peripheral primitive neuroectodermal tumour which have now become collectively referred to as the Ewing sarcoma family of tumours (EFT). The vast majority of EFT is characterised by a fusion transcript involving *EWSR1* fused in approximately 85% of cases with an *ETS* gene family member, the most common partner is *FLi1*. The rare variants and those with non-*ETS* fusion transcript are listed in **Table 4.2**. More recently, it has been shown that some cases of Ewing sarcoma have a more pleomorphic morphology than previously recognised, and that approximately two thirds of the *EWSR1*-negative EFT harbour a fusion gene *BCOR-CCNB3* and *BCOR-CCNB3* and *CIC-DUX4* (**Table 4.2**) [27,28].

Phosphaturic mesenchymal tumour

This is an exceptionally rare tumour that occurs both in bone and soft tissue. The majority of patients have long-standing osteomalacia that is resistant to calcium and vitamin D treatment. Histologically, the tumour presents with a wide range of histological features (**Figure 4.6**) and can be diagnostically challenging. The tumour, even when it is too small to be detected clinically, may produce large amounts of fibroblastic growth factor 23 (FGF23) causing the systemic paraneoplastic osteomalacic syndrome.

FGF23 plays a key role in phosphate homeostasis, and the main source of this protein under physiological conditions is bone cells (osteocytes and osteoblasts). Removal of the tumour results in a dramatic drop in the circulating levels of FGF23, and reversal of the

Table 4.2 Translocations involving the EWSR1 gene	
Tumour type	**EWSR1 and partner genes**
Ewing sarcoma	EWSR1 - ETS (common variants): *EWSR1-FLI1* *EWSR1-ERG*
	EWSR1 - ETS (rare variants): *EWSR1-ETV1* *EWSR1-ETV4* *EWSR1-FEV*
	EWSR1 - non ETS (rare variants): *EWSR1-NFATc2* *EWSR1-POU5F1* *EWSR1-SMARCA5* *EWSR1-PATZ* *EWSR1-SP3*
Rarely occurring in bone	
Angiomatoid fibrous histiocytoma	*EWSR1-ATF1*
	EWSR1-CREB1
Clear cell sarcoma	*EWSR1-CREB1*
Desmoplastic small round cell tumour	*EWSR1-WT1*
Extraskeletal mesenchymal chondrosarcoma	*EWSR1-NR4A3*
Mixed tumour/myoepithelioma	*EWSR1-POU5F1*
	EWSR1-PBX1
Odontogenic* clear cell carcinoma and hyalinising clear cell carcinoma of salivary origin	*EWSR1-ATF1*
Non-ETS family is shown in blue. *Odontogenic tumours occur in bone	

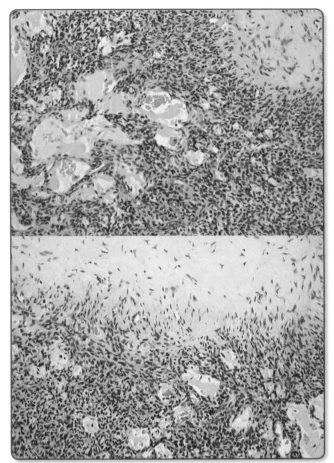

Figure 4.6 A photomicrograph of a phosphaturic mesenchymal tumour showing bland spindle cells set in a highly vascular background with nodular hyalinised areas.

osteomalacia. In addition to using the aberrantly high levels of expression of FGF23 for reaching a diagnosis, serial measurements of calcium and phosphate or circulating FGF23 can be employed to monitor disease recurrence. At a tissue level, antibodies to FGF23 do not provide sufficient specificity to be useful in the clinical setting, and gene expression detected by RT-PCR, although highly sensitive, is not adequately specific as some other tumours (ABC and chondromyxoid fibroma) and produce low levels of FGF23. Andrew Folpe's group reported that the novel chromogenic in situ hybridisation technique could be used successfully for detection of *FGF23* messenger RNA, using formalin-fixed paraffin-embedded tissue [29]. The RNA-SCOPE technology obviates the difficulties encountered with immunohistochemistry and RT-PCR.

Recently, an *FN1-FGFR1* gene fusion has been described in approximately 60% of these tumours [30].

Pseudomyogenic haemangioendothelioma

This is an unusual tumour that can occur in a range of sites including subcutaneous tissue, deep soft tissue and bone. This tumour behaves in an indolent fashion that rarely metastasises but is often multifocal [31,32]. The rarity of this tumour along with the unusual morphology comprising epithelioid and myogenic-type appearance and immunohistochemical findings (cytokeratin, CD31 and ERG immunoreactive) can lead to misdiagnoses. The recently reported *SERPINE1-FOSB* fusion gene that is characteristic of this neoplasm will allow robust diagnoses [33].

Epithelioid haemangioma of bone

This is a locally aggressive tumour characterised by numerous blood vessels lined by plump endothelial cells with epithelioid morphology set in a fibrous stroma with an eosinophil-rich mixed inflammatory infiltrate. The tumour has a multilobular growth pattern and host bone permeation can be seen. Up to 25% of the cases are multifocal.

A *ZFP36-FOSB* fusion has been reported in epithelioid haemangioma (EH) with atypical histological features [34]. Subsequently, a *FOS* gene rearrangement was identified in 29% of EH. However, when the cohort was restricted to bone, 59% of the intraosseous EH demonstrated a *FOS* gene rearrangement [35].

Key points for clinical practice

- Before reporting a case review all clinical information particularly look at previous histology and ensure that the relevant imaging is reviewed by a specialist musculoskeletal radiologist before providing a diagnosis.
- It is rare for a diagnosis of a `round cell tumour' to be provided today. In the absence of an Ewing rearrangement being identified, look for a BCOR-CCNB3 and a CIC-DUX4 fusion transcript.
- A significant number of bone tumours can be classified on the basis of molecular genetic alterations.
- There is a wide range of tumours, other than Ewing sarcoma, which harbour an EWSR1 fusion gene.
- A significant number of osteoclast-rich lesions can be classified by a genetic alteration. In the absence of a H3F3 mutation, be cautious of making a diagnosis of a giant cell tumour of bone.
- Rarely a H3F3 alteration is detected in malignant bone and soft tissue tumours.
- GNAS1 mutations can be detected in the majority of the cases of fibrous dysplasia but this alteration is not detected in parosteal osteosarcoma.

REFERENCES

1. Bovee JV, Cleton-Jansen AM, Wuyts W, et al. EXT-mutation analysis and loss of heterozygosity in sporadic and hereditary osteochondromas and secondary chondrosarcomas. Am J Hum Genet 1999; 65:689–698.
2. Amary MF, Bacsi K, Maggiani F, et al. IDH1 and IDH2 mutations are frequent events in central chondrosarcoma and central and periosteal chondromas but not in other mesenchymal tumours. J Pathol 2011; 224:334–343.
3. Damato S, Alorjani M, Bonar F, et al. IDH1 mutations are not found in cartilaginous tumours other than central and periosteal chondrosarcomas and enchondromas. Histopathology 2012; 60:363–365.
4. Amary MF, Ye H, Forbes G, et al. Isocitrate dehydrogenase 1 mutations (IDH1) and p16/CDKN2A copy number change in conventional chondrosarcomas. Virchows Arch 2015; 466:217–222.

5. Guilhamon P, Eskandarpour M, Halai D, et al. Meta-analysis of IDH-mutant cancers identifies EBF1 as an interaction partner for TET2. Nat Commun 2013; 4:2166.
6. Tarpey PS, Behjati S, Cooke SL, et al. Frequent mutation of the major cartilage collagen gene COL2A1 in chondrosarcoma. Nat Genet 2013; 45:923–926.
7. Pansuriya TC, Kroon HM, Bovee JV. Enchondromatosis: insights on the different subtypes. Int J Clin Exp Pathol 2010; 3:557–569.
8. Amary MF, Damato S, Halai D, et al. Ollier disease and Maffucci syndrome are caused by somatic mosaic mutations of IDH1 and IDH2. Nat Genet 2011; 43:1262–1265.
9. Pansuriya TC, van Eijk R, d'Adamo P, et al. Somatic mosaic IDH1 and IDH2 mutations are associated with enchondroma and spindle cell hemangioma in Ollier disease and Maffucci syndrome. Nat Genet 2011; 43:1256–1261.
10. Parsons DW, Jones S, Zhang X, et al. An integrated genomic analysis of human glioblastoma multiforme. Science 2008; 321:1807–1812.
11. Schumacher T, Bunse L, Pusch S, et al. A vaccine targeting mutant IDH1 induces antitumour immunity. Nature 2014; 512:324–327.
12. Rohle D, Popovici-Muller J, Palaskas N, et al. An inhibitor of mutant IDH1 delays growth and promotes differentiation of glioma cells. Science 2013; 340:626–630.
13. Wang L, Motoi T, Khanin R, et al. Identification of a novel, recurrent HEY1-NCOA2 fusion in mesenchymal chondrosarcoma based on a genome-wide screen of exon-level expression data. Genes Chromosomes Cancer 2012; 51:127–139.
14. Nord KH, Lilljebjorn H, Vezzi F, et al. GRM1 is upregulated through gene fusion and promoter swapping in chondromyxoid fibroma. Nat Genet 2014; 46:474–477.
15. Oliveira AM, Perez-Atayde AR, Inwards CY, et al. USP6 and CDH11 oncogenes identify the neoplastic cell in primary aneurysmal bone cysts and are absent in so-called secondary aneurysmal bone cysts. Am J Pathol 2004; 165:1773–1780.
16. Behjati S, Tarpey PS, Presneau N, et al. Distinct H3F3A and H3F3B driver mutations define chondroblastoma and giant cell tumor of bone. Nat Genet 2013; 45:1479–1482.
17. Presneau N, Baumhoer D, Behjati S, et al. Diagnostic value of H3F3A mutations in giant cell tumour of bone compared to osteoclast-rich mimics. J Pathol: Clin Res 2015; 1:113–123.
18. Kato Kaneko M, Liu X, Oki H, et al. Isocitrate dehydrogenase mutation is frequently observed in giant cell tumor of bone. Cancer Sci 2014; 105:744–748.
19. Erickson-Johnson MR, Chou MM, Evers BR, et al. Nodular fasciitis: a novel model of transient neoplasia induced by MYH9-USP6 gene fusion. Lab Invest 2011; 91:1427–1433.
20. Fletcher CDM, World Health Organization, International Agency for Research on Cancer. WHO classification of tumours of soft tissue and bone, 4th edn. Lyon: IARC Press, 2013:468.
21. Agaram NP, LeLoarer FV, Zhang L, et al. USP6 gene rearrangements occur preferentially in giant cell reparative granulomas of the hands and feet but not in gnathic location. Hum Pathol 2014; 45:1147–1152.
22. Flanagan AM, Speight PM. Giant cell lesions of the craniofacial bones. Head Neck Pathol 2014; 8:445–453.
23. Fernanda Amary M, Ye H, Berisha F, et al. Fibroblastic growth factor receptor 1 amplification in osteosarcoma is associated with poor response to neo-adjuvant chemotherapy. Cancer Med 2014; 3:980–987.
24. Idowu BD, Al-Adnani M, O'Donnell P, et al. A sensitive mutation-specific screening technique for GNAS1 mutations in cases of fibrous dysplasia: the first report of a codon 227 mutation in bone. Histopathology 2007; 50:691–704.
25. Carter JM, Inwards CY, Jin L, et al. Activating GNAS mutations in parosteal osteosarcoma. Am J Surg Pathol 2014; 38:402–409.
26. Salinas-Souza C, De Andrea C, Bihl M, et al. GNAS mutations are not detected in parosteal and low-grade central osteosarcomas. Mod Pathol 2015; 28:1336–1342.
27. Antonescu C. Round cell sarcomas beyond Ewing: emerging entities. Histopathology 2014; 64:26–37.
28. Marino-Enriquez A, Fletcher CD. Round cell sarcomas – biologically important refinements in subclassification. Int J Biochem Cell Biol 2014; 53:493–504.
29. Carter JM, Caron BL, Dogan A, et al. A novel chromogenic in situ hybridization assay for FGF23 mRNA in phosphaturic mesenchymal tumors. Am J Surg Pathol 2015; 39:75–83.
30. Lee JC, Jeng YM, Su SY, et al. Identification of a novel FN1-FGFR1 genetic fusion as a frequent event in phosphaturic mesenchymal tumour. J Pathol 2015; 235:539–545.
31. Hornick JL, Fletcher CD. Pseudomyogenic hemangioendothelioma: a distinctive, often multicentric tumor with indolent behavior. Am J Surg Pathol 2011; 35:190–201.

32. Amary MF, O'Donnell P, Berisha F, et al. Pseudomyogenic (epithelioid sarcoma-like) hemangioendothelioma: characterization of five cases. Skeletal Radiol 2013; 42:947–957.
33. Walther C, Tayebwa J, Lilljebjorn H, et al. A novel SERPINE1-FOSB fusion gene results in transcriptional up-regulation of FOSB in pseudomyogenic haemangioendothelioma. J Pathol 2014; 232:534–540.
34. Antonescu CR, Chen HW, Zhang L, et al. ZFP36-FOSB fusion defines a subset of epithelioid hemangioma with atypical features. Genes Chromosomes Cancer 2014; 53:951–959.
35. Huang SC, Zhang L, Sung YS, et al. Frequent FOS gene rearrangements in epithelioid hemangioma: a molecular study of 58 cases with morphologic reappraisal. Am J Surg Pathol 2015; 39:1313–1321.

Chapter 5

Post-mortem computed tomography and its application in autopsies

Guy N Rutty, Bruno Morgan

INTRODUCTION

The invasive autopsy has been considered the gold standard for investigating the cause of death for thousands of years. More recently, practitioners and researchers have sought alternatives to minimise, if not remove, the necessity for this procedure [1]. This has been driven by two objectives: firstly, the desire to improve the quality, speed, cost and efficiency of the investigation, and secondly, possibly more importantly, a perceived dislike of invasive autopsies by the general public and medical profession, and the requirements of some religious doctrines and law [2]. Although several non-invasive and so-called minimally invasive alternatives have been described in the scientific and general literature, to date no imaging alternative has been widely accepted as equal to or better than the invasive examination. However, we believe that there is a true alternative to the traditional invasive autopsy, one that is being promoted now within the literature as a key development in the accurate investigation of death for both adults and children; post-mortem cross-sectional imaging [4].

This chapter provides a brief synopsis of the current state of practice of adult post-mortem cross-sectional imaging and specifically post-mortem computed tomography (PMCT). We also describe how it can be used in coronial autopsy practice, as an adjunct or replacement to the traditional invasive autopsy.

Terminology

It is important to use consistent terminology when discussing any subject in medicine. For example, a number of terms have been introduced to describe the same process of imaging investigation, including 'virtual autopsy,' 'digital autopsy' and Virtopsy. This diversity can be misleading, especially if the term does not specifically describe the processes involved. In an attempt to standardise terminology, a group of international experts have put forward a proposed system of nomenclature [5]. Using the baseline terminology of post-mortem cross-sectional imaging to distinguish this from other forms of medical imaging, the group

Guy N Rutty MBE MD MBBS FRCPath DipRCPath (forensic) FCSFS FFFLM AFHEA, East Midlands Forensic Pathology Unit, University of Leicester, Leicester UK. Email: gnr3@le.ac.uk (for correspondence)

Bruno Morgan PhD BM BCh MRCP FRCR, Radiology Department, University of Leicester, Leicester Royal Infirmary, Leicester UK

suggested the adoption of two core terms based upon the type of imaging modality used: post-mortem computed tomography, (PMCT) and post-mortem magnetic resonance (PMMR). This chapter will refer to adult PMCT only.

The term PMCT describes a so-called native scan, i.e. a scan with no additional procedures. This is the only truly non-invasive form of PMCT. Scans can be 'enhanced' where at least one extra procedure is undertaken to assist diagnostic interpretation of the images. This will usually involve an invasive procedure, such as the use of angiography (e.g. PMCT angiography or PMCTA), pulmonary ventilation, or needle biopsy. Care must be taken when explaining these procedures to relatives, lay people and even medical professionals, who are not familiar with these techniques to make sure they understand what procedures will be performed on the body. Therefore, we suggest that the term 'minimally-invasive' is used rather than 'non-invasive' if extra procedures are used.

A BRIEF HISTORICAL OVERVIEW

Radiology has been a part of investigations into cause of death since its first use in a homicide investigation in England in 1896 [6]. It has principally been limited to forensic practice, particularly for the investigation of fire- and projectile-related deaths and child deaths. The first documented use of computed tomography (CT) in clinical forensic practice was in 1977 for the investigation of cranial ballistic injury [7]. This was followed in 1983 with the first reported use of PMCT for the investigation of an underwater diving-related death [8]. Although these early pioneers realised the potential of PMCT within autopsy practice, it was not until 1994 that it was first reported from Israel that PMCT could be used both as an adjunct and as an alternative to conventional adult autopsy [9]. This was followed in 1996, when a group from the UK proposed the use of magnetic resonance imaging as an alternative for perinatal autopsies [10].

After a slow start, the number of scientific publications began to increase in 2003, particularly with the work of the Virtopsy group [11]. Technology was changing with the development of faster and more powerful CT scanners and image processing software. Over the last decade, we have seen the global introduction of PMCT and PMMR into adult and child autopsy practice, with an associated increase in supporting research and literature [12]. Scanners have been placed into mortuaries to facilitate diagnostic services [13], as well as having been adopted into temporary mortuaries for mass fatality investigations (MFI) [14]. In 2012, the International Society for Forensic Radiology and Imaging (ISFRI) was founded along with the first dedicated autopsy imaging journal; Journal of Forensic Radiology and Imaging to promote further, advise upon and expand the use of post-mortem cross-sectional imaging and, through their working groups and annual conferences, have provided a number of international positional statements. In the United Kingdom, the Department of Health published a visionary document in 2012 considering the introduction of a PMCT-based national autopsy service [15]. Unfortunately, to date this visionary document's content has not been realised.

PMCT

Who, where, when and how

Who, where, when and by what means a person came by their death (usually simplified to 'how') are the core questions to be addressed by a medicolegal autopsy. The emphasis on which of these questions needs to be addressed varies from case to case. For example, if a family member collapses at a known time within the home, 'how' becomes the principle question, whereas an unidentified body discovered in a field will probably require all four questions to be answered. For a mass fatality incident, the cause of death may be all too clear and 'who' the victims were is paramount for both legal and family reasons.

PMCT can be used in two ways to consider these questions – to complement the findings from invasive autopsy or as an alternative. In both approaches, PMCT can inform who, when and how but rarely where. However, the invasive autopsy may also be unhelpful as regards where a person died, which is often better decided by a thorough external examination of the body and the site where it was found. As the external examination of the body remains an integral part of a PMCT examination, replacing the invasive autopsy with PMCT does not compromise the consideration of where the person died.

Who

The use of radiology in human cadaver identification was first reported in 1972 by Culbert and Law [16]. By comparing the unique biological features of nasal accessory and mastoid sinuses on ante- and post-mortem radiographs they were able to confirm the identity of a deceased individual. Radiography established a role for mass fatality examinations in 1949 when it was used to help identify the 119 victims of the Great Lakes liner 'Noronic' disaster in Toronto, Canada [17]. In these cases, radiology provided a positive identification for 24 of the most severely disfigured bodies.

In around 2004, Rutty suggested that a mobile CT scanner could be used at a scene or temporary mortuary of a mass fatality incident. Although the use of mobile PMCT in a medicolegal autopsy setting was first reported in Japan [18], it was not until 2006 that Rutty et al reported the use of mobile PMCT at a multiple fatality incident (MFIs) [19]. The Leicester research group went on to report a teleradiology system for remote data reporting in MFIs, which they termed the FiMAG system [20]. PMCT's potential for use in Disaster Victim Identification (DVI) has also been considered by the Virtopsy group who illustrated its ability to collect information to complete the Interpol DVI forms and suggested the use of a remotely operated robotic sampling system for contaminated incidents [21,22]. Since then, PMCT has been utilised in MFIs in military conflict areas; the 2009 bush fires in Victoria, Australia [23]; the Norwegian shootings and more recently the MH17 air crash.

ISFRI have endorsed the use of PMCT for mass fatality investigation [24,25]. A review of the most regularly used anthropological identification techniques, by Brough et al [26] demonstrated that all the measurements and morphological features required for these methods can be extracted from PMCT data. In a more recent publication, the same authors also considered the use of PMCT for odontological identification purposes [27], developed a minimum dataset approach for PMCT-assisted identification [28] (**Figure 5.1**) and suggested that it would also be possible to complete the majority of the current DVI Interpol form using only PMCT, with an external examination [29]. These publications illustrate how PMCT could be used for identification purposes, highlighting its potential to provide information with regard to personal effects, clothing, external and internal biological features as well as being used for osteological and odontological identification purposes. When used in conjunction with an external examination PMCT has the potential to facilitate the identification of single or multiple fatalities.

When

The estimation of the time since death, also known as the 'post-mortem interval' (PMI), can be attempted by a variety of methods [30]. As a number of post-mortem changes can be observed with time with PMCT, these changes could be used to estimate a time since death although this area of research is currently in its infancy. The following PMCT-related changes have been described with regard to estimating a PMI.

Livor mortis

Shiotani et al in 2002 were the first to report that hypostasis (lividity, livor mortis) could be observed by PMCT within 2 hours of death as a high-density fluid level in the lumen of the heart and great vessels (**Figure 5.2**). They proposed that this appearance was caused by the gravitational separation of serum and red cells following the cessation of blood flow [31]. This post-mortem change has now also been reported in the veins, organs and tissues. In the cranium, it occurs within the posterior sagittal sinus, straight sinus and transvers sinus, where it can be mistaken by the unwary as acute thrombosis or as subarachnoid haemorrhage [32–34] (**Figure 5.3**). It does not occur in everyone, being influenced by factors such as age, clinical anaemia, blood volume, position after death and temperature. Hypostasis is seen in the lungs as increased attenuation, and occurs between the dependent and nondependent aspects. In the skin, increased attenuation occurs between the subcutaneous fat and dermis, with the dermis becoming thicker in the dependent parts of the body compared to the nondependent parts.

Vascular wall changes

One of the changes that can be observed with a native PMCT scan after death is that the great vessels collapse. A number of authors have published observations related to aortic collapse at different anatomical sites with time [35–37] (**Figure 5.4**). These changes may be affected by the physical build of the deceased, cardiopulmonary resuscitation (CPR), haemorrhage and decomposition.

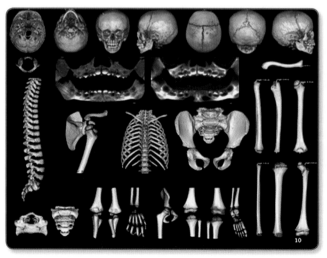

Figure 5.1 An example of the dataset used for osteological and odontological assessment for identification purposes as described by Brough et al [28]. Courtesy of Dr A Brough, East Midlands Forensic Pathology Unit, University of Leicester, UK.

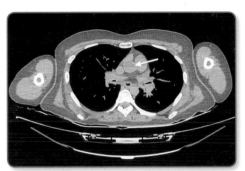

Figure 5.2 Axial section of the thorax showing post-mortem blood hypostasis level (arrow) within the thoracic aorta.

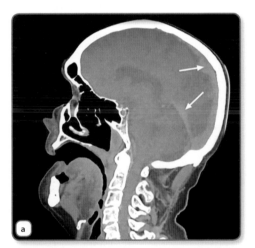

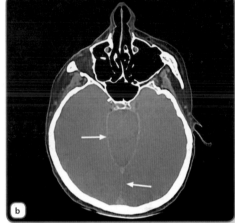

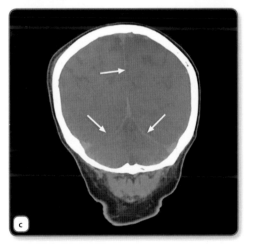

Figure 5.3 (a) Sagittal, (b) axial and (c) coronal sections of the head showing post-mortem blood hypostasis (arrows) mimicking subarchnoid haemorrhage.

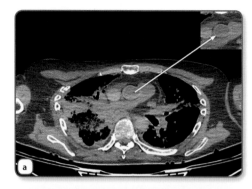
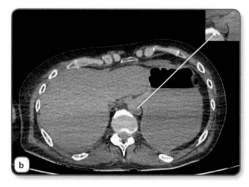

Figure 5.4 (a) Post-mortem collapse of the ascending aorta, (b) abdominal aorta at emergence through diaphragm and (c) abdominal aorta close to bifurcation into iliac vessels varies depending upon the anatomical position in the body.

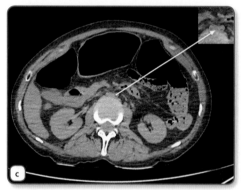

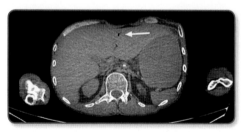

Figure 5.5 Axial image showing air (arrow) in the portal veins as an early postmortem change.

Post-mortem gas formation

Following death the first site of true putrefactive gas production is generally observed by PMCT within the intestinal wall and mesenteric and portal venous systems [34] (**Figure 5.5**). It then develops within all vascular spaces and potential anatomical spaces. However not all gas seen by PMCT is due to decomposition. Shiotani et al described a relationship between gastrointestinal distension attributed to CPR and the presence of hepatic portal venous gas observed within 2 hours of death [38]. Other authors have reported similar observations [39–43].

Thyroid gland changes

A study by Ishida et al reports changes in the thyroid gland from ante-mortem CT (AMCT) to PMCT, which correlated with the interval from death [44]. However, they concluded that these data could not be used to predict accurately the time of death.

Cerebral parenchyma attenuation

After death, blurring and loss of definition of the grey-white matter junction, a decrease in cerebral attenuation and sulci effacement is observed early with PMCT with complete loss of grey-white matter differentiation seen within 2–3 days after death [34]. It has been suggested that changes in the density of the deep white matter tracts of the brain correlate well with interval from death, and this may be used to help predict time of death [45; W Klein, 2014, personal communication].

How

The use of PMCT to complement a full or limited invasive autopsy has been suggested as the new gold standard [46]. It can be used in the following ways:

- To screen for potentially hazardous items in or outside the body, and the presence of infectious diseases such as tuberculosis [47].
- To examine areas of the body not normally examined at autopsy [48].
- To avoid disfiguring procedures such as facial dissection for orbital fractures [49].
- To plan the retrieval of evidential objects such as projectiles from the body.
- To consider and demonstrate projectile and penetrating weapon paths through body cavities.
- To determine whether specialist autopsy procedures are required, e.g. to confirm the presence of a cardiac air embolus [50].
- To illustrate skeletal trauma in greater detail than an autopsy provides (**Figure 5.6**).
- To provide a permanent record of the pre-autopsied body.
- To provide images of the body for court purposes. 'Sanitised' still or video reconstructions can be presented to the court, particularly in trauma, suspicious or homicide deaths.

For some, replacing the invasive autopsy with PMCT remains a step too far [3]. For example, in traumatic or suspicious deaths the police and courts are likely to still expect

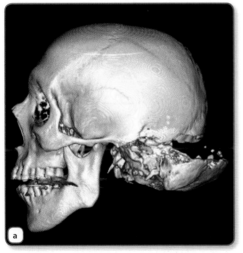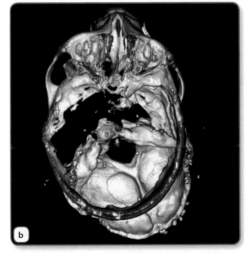

Figure 5.6 (a) Sagittal and (b) axial image of cranial injuries sustained by a motor cyclist wearing a full face helmet at the time of the incident illustrating how post-mortem computed tomography can be used to consider skeletal head injuries. Courtesy of Dr A Brough, East Midlands Forensic Pathology Unit, University of Leicester, UK.

an invasive autopsy, although this is due to a reluctance by the criminal justice service to adopt new legal processes rather than any specific limitation of PMCT [46]. However, there is growing scientific evidence to support the transition from invasive autopsy to PMCT, and professional bodies in the UK, such as the Royal Colleges of Radiologists and Pathologists, have endorsed PMCT as a replacement in certain circumstances [51]. Conversely, in Japan where the national autopsy percentage is in single figures, PMCT has been adopted as a means of increasing their rate of post-mortem investigation without the need for invasive procedures. To the author's knowledge, however, they are currently the only country to have a national post-mortem cross-sectional imaging service.

One key problem to be addressed if PMCT is to be used as a replacement for the invasive autopsy is the accurate diagnosis of coronary artery disease, the most common form of sudden unexpected natural death in the UK. Fatal haemorrhages, such as subarachnoid haemorrhage, haemorrhagic stroke, haemopericardium and abdominal aortic rupture, are readily diagnosed using unenhanced PMCT (**Figure 5.7**). As for clinical imaging, however, assessment of coronary artery luminal pathological abnormalities, which account for 80% of medicolegal natural deaths, requires some form of image enhancement using injected contrast media. Even with injected contrast media the diagnosis of pulmonary thromboembolus, respiratory disease and gastrointestinal haemorrhage may be difficult if it is not directly suggested by the person's medical history. This can explain disappointing results when the findings of unenhanced PMCT are compared with autopsy results [52]. However, these data do not take into account the circumstances of death and if an

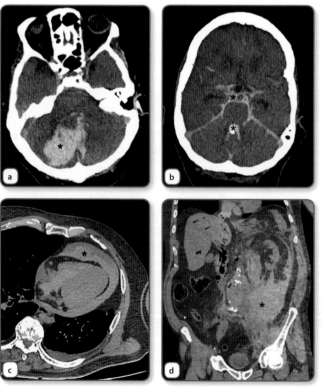

Figure 5.7 (a) Axial image of a haemorrhagic infarct (*) affecting the right lobe of the cerebellum. (b) Axial cranial image showing a subarachnoid haemorrhage (*). (c) Axial image of the heart showing a haemopericardium (*). (d) Coronal image of the abdomen showing a ruptured abdominal aortic aneurysm (*).

assessment is made purely on clinical history alone, or if the assessor simply guesses ischaemic heart disease in all cases, the correct cause of death will be determined in 80% of cases [53,54].

PMCTA

To overcome this inherent problem with unenhanced native PMCT, three different approaches to visualising the vasculature of the cadaver have been developed; so-called PMCTA [55]. By using one of these approaches (depending on operator, clinical circumstances and country of use), it is possible to visualise the lumen of the coronary arteries. This is arguably in more detail than can be seen at autopsy, and thus PMCT becomes comparable for the diagnosis of stenotic coronary artery disease. Despite this, specific plaque pathology remains occult to PMCTA, and other imaging systems, such as optical coherence tomography, may be required [56,57]. PMCTA also offers the opportunity to study myocardial and valvular pathology but the accuracy of diagnosis is as yet unclear.

Whole body PMCTA

In 2005, Jackowski et al described a technique of whole body PMCTA using a roller pump and meglumine-iothalamate as a contrast agent [58]. Although this water soluble contrast agent solution provided excellent vessel visualisation, it caused tissue oedema and histological artefacts. This was overcome by using polyethylene glycol as a solvent [59]. The University Centre of Legal Medicine in Lausanne, Switzerland, has developed the contrast agent and delivery method into the technique known as MPMCTA (Multiphase Post-mortem Computed Tomography Angiography). This technique uses a perfusion device (Virtangio, Fumedica AG, Sz) with an oily contrast agent mixture (Angiofil, Fumedica AG, Sz) in paraffin oil [60]. The standard protocol of MPMCTA consists of one native CT scan followed by the cannulation of the femoral vessels of one side of the body. During the cannulation process, blood samples are collected for toxicological and biochemical analysis. A contrast mixture of 6% Angiofil and paraffin oil (paraffinum liquidum) is then infused, first into the femoral artery (arterial phase) and then into the femoral vein (venous phase) and finally further arterial contrast is injected with 'venting' from the vein to give a 'dynamic phase' image acquisition. By using whole body PMCTA the whole vascular system of the head, thorax, and abdomen is visualised with the exceptions of the cerebral sinus and vessels, which may be occluded by large post-mortem clots (**Figure 5.8**).

Targeted PMCTA

Targeted PMCTA, unlike whole body PMCTA, is specifically designed to target the coronary arteries and left heart valves and chambers. The technique often shows the great veins, right heart and arteries within the thoracic cavity as well. Developed independently by two different centres in the UK, the technique places a urinary balloon catheter into the aorta just above the aortic valve to facilitate the injection of positive (Urografin) and negative (air) contrast mediums into the coronary arteries [61,62]. Although the contrast agents can be delivered by hand injection, the use of an automatic injection pump 'dynamically' during scanning allows for better imaging of the coronary arteries [63] (**Figure 5.9**).

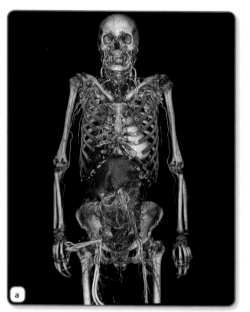
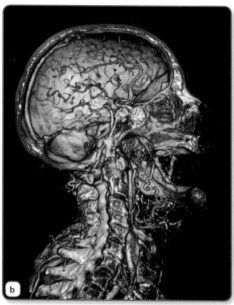

Figure 5.8 (a, b) Examples of whole body multislice post-mortem CT angiography to illustrate the degree of visualisation of the vascular tree and organs that are possible using this technique. Courtesy of Dr A Brough, East Midlands Forensic Pathology Unit, University of Leicester, UK.

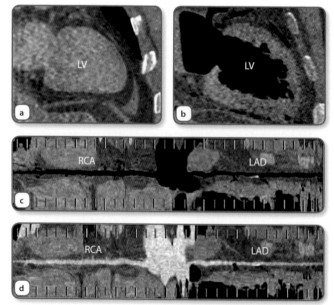

Figure 5.9 (a) The left ventricle (LV) seen with a native, nonenhanced scan. The chamber cannot be seen. The chamber, however, is opened up with an enhanced scan (b) using air as the negative contrast agent. The examination of both the left anterior descending (LAD) and right coronary arteries (RCA) using (c) air as a negative contrast agent and (d) urograffin as a positive agent (curved multiplanar reformation).

Chest compression PMCTA

Sakamoto et al and Iizuka K et al described a third form of PMCTA; chest compression PMCTA [64,65]. Chest compressions during cardiopulmonary resuscitation generate a cardiac output of approximately one-fourth the normal state and this can be used to generate sufficient circulation for PMCTA. Contrast media can be injected into an arm vein and through cadaveric chest compression, it can enter the right atrium move through the heart and lungs to reach the aorta, and then go into the arterial tree including the proximal portions of the cerebral, coronary, celiac, superior mesenteric arteries, etc. This form of PMCTA is usually performed within 3 hours after death to avoid problems associated with increasing post-mortem vascular permeability.

VENTILATED PMCT

In clinical practice, radiography and CT of the thorax is ideally performed in inspiration and breath-hold. 'Expiratory' images may be used in addition to look at pulmonary dynamics, but an 'expiratory' image is not ideal on its own due to crowding of pulmonary vessels, areas of atelectasis and 'dependent' changes of airspace collapse and fluid, making interstitial or nodular changes less apparent [66,67]. In many ways, a post-mortem CT scan mimics a clinical CT scan in expiratory phase, but in addition they may show obscuration of lung pathology due to an increase in pulmonary opacification caused by livor mortis (**Figure 5.10**). The rapid onset of this early post-mortem change may obscure true ante-mortem lung pathology and could be mistaken for aspiration, pulmonary oedema or pneumonia by the unwary [68].

In an attempt to overcome this problem, Germerott et al developed a method of ventilated PMCT (VPMCT) [69]. They have described the use of a portable home care ventilator, which delivers ventilation by a continuous positive airway pressure (CPAP)-mask (or endotracheal tube or a laryngeal mask if present from previous medical care). Although clinical ventilation uses continuous pressures of between 5 cm H_2O and 20 cm H_2O to avoid lung damage that may occur at higher pressures [70,71], they found a higher pressure of 40 cm H_2O was required to unfold the cadaver lung. No lung damage was apparent on PMCT at this higher pressure. They showed this system could produce significant lung expansion and it would improve diagnostic ability (**Figure 5.10**), including wound track pathology for penetrating trauma to the lung. They also reported a number of potential problems including difficult air delivery due to the presence of rigor mortis to the jaw, movement artefact caused by their method of ventilation, gastric air dilation as well as poor lung expansion in the presence of pre-existing pneumothorax or haemothorax [72,73].

Building upon this initial work Robinson et al reported the use of a supraglottic airway and a clinical portable ventilator to deliver CPAP at 40 cm H_2O to mimic clinical breath-hold inspiratory scans [74]. This method provides a rapid form of VPMCT allowing for the post-mortem radiological comparison of native (expiratory) and inspiratory phase imaging. However, similar to the method of Germerott et al, this technique may suffer from air leakage and gastric dilatation if a good laryngeal seal is not achieved. To overcome this, Rutty et al described methods for inserting a cuffed airway, either endotracheal tube or a tube via a tracheostomy. They suggest an algorithm to aid choice of method, including the presence of jaw rigor, but recognise the choice of method depends on the context, operator and their ethical and religious environment. They showed that adequate cadaver lung expansion can be achieved for all methods, but they favoured the use of a modified endotracheal tube inserted through the cricothyroid membrane. They found that the technique could be taught to nonmedical personnel, such as anatomical pathology technologists or radiographers [75].

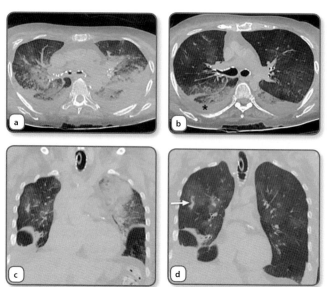

Figure 5.10 Axial and coronal PMCT images, pre (a and c) and post (b and d) ventilation in a road traffic death. The preventilation images show a combination of haemorrhage, post-mortem lividity and dependent atelectasis. The postventilation images more closely resemble clinical scans and show clearing of post-mortem changes, but the haemothorax (*) and pulmonary contusions (arrow) remain.

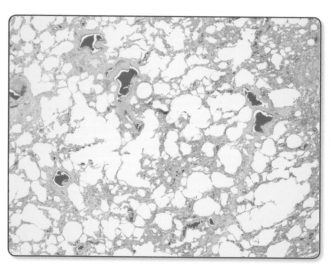

Figure 5.11 The appearance of the lungs post ventilated post-mortem computed tomography (VPMCT). Note the over distended appearance of the alveoli caused by VPMCT. Haematoxylin and eosin stain with 1.25´ objective lens. Courtesy of Dr M Biggs, East Midlands Forensic Pathology Unit, University of Leicester, UK.

Currently there is no scientific evidence that shows that enhanced imaging of the lungs is required to diagnose the presence of pathology in the dead, and at the time of the writing of this chapter very few centres in the world use anything other than a native scan for the diagnosis of natural thoracic disease and trauma. Our experience is that VPMCT does not affect the subsequent macroscopic examination of the lungs at autopsy, but histological examination of the post-ventilated pulmonary parenchyma is affected; the alveoli appear over distended similar to those seen with terminal clinical ventilation or following CPR with the use of a definitive airway (**Figure 5.11**). Whether this change affects the ability to diagnose ante-mortem lung pathology, such as emphysema or due to drowning, remains to be seen.

BIOPSY PMCT

Histology may be required in post-mortem investigation, although the necessity to undertake such examination has been debated within the published literature [76–80]. Currently, there are no guidelines to the author's knowledge as to when tissue sampling could be used to support imaging findings alone.

If tissue sampling for histological diagnosis or tissue retrieval for other diagnostic tests, such as the investigation of drowning using bacterioplankton PCR probes [81], is performed it is therefore ideal to use a minimally invasive approach, especially as the major aim of PMCT is to reduce the incisions to the body to a minimum.

Needle biopsy in association with autopsy practice was first reported in 1955 with a number of studies reported in the literature since then [82]. In clinical radiology tissue samples, including cutting needle core biopsies, are routinely taken using CT to guide the needle. In 2007, the Virtopsy group reported the acquisition of post-mortem histological material using fluoroscopic multislice CT to guide the needle [83]. They were concerned that using CT fluoroscopic techniques (where the CT scanner is used to obtain 'real-time' images during the procedure) would result in high exposures of ionising radiation to staff. To avoid this in clinical practice, radiation protective shields or aprons are worn. Also the operator will often use a 'sequential' rather than 'real-time' scanning approach, leaving the room between scans and advancing the needle incrementally between scans, based on image geometry and experience. For clinical biopsies, the needle must not only hit the desired target, but also miss important structures that may be in the way, so the biopsy is normally performed by a highly trained member of staff and may be time consuming. However, as the actual needle path is of less importance in the post-mortem setting, the Virtopsy group have developed robotic systems for histological sampling with remote targeting (telebiopsy), which does not require an image interpretation expert to be present in the scanner [83–88]. This work has culminated to date in the aspirational Virtobot 2.0 system with its robotic sampling system.

LABORATORY TESTS AND PMCT

A proportion of autopsies will require additional laboratory tests, e.g. toxicology, microbiology, biochemistry, metabolic or genetic studies. The need for these tests can often be predicted from the clinical history and therefore appropriate authority can be sought and retrieval during the autopsy can be planned in advance (e.g. DNA where the identity is unknown). However, the need for such tests may only become apparent during the autopsy examination.

Tissue and biological fluid samples can be readily obtained for laboratory and identification purposes using PMCT, so the need of such samples should be considered in advance. PMCT can be used to guide samples from any part of the body as described in the biopsy section above. DNA identification samples are not affected by both targeted and whole body PMCTA [89]. Targeted coronary PMCTA has been shown in one series not to affect toxicology and biochemistry laboratory tests [90], but multiphase PMCTA, using oily contrast media is reported to affect subsequent laboratory tests, depending on the sample type [91–93]. Therefore ideally, sampling should be done before any contrast agent is used that may affect any subsequent sampling.

Organ and tissue retrieval

The authors support organ and tissue retrieval for transplantation purposes from the dead. As organs must be retrieved in <5 minutes after the cessation of a circulation then PMCT will not conflict with this procedure. Enhanced systems such as PMCTA and VPMCT may be problematic if there has been surgical removal of vital organs or key blood vessels. For cadaveric skin and bone tissue retrieval is less problematic as viable tissue is less scarce. Although there is no proven risk from the use of nonsterile contrast medium it is probably best avoided if there is a likelihood of tissue retrieval.

Key points for clinical practice

- Post-mortem cross sectional imaging is recognised throughout the world as both an adjunct to, if not a replacement to the traditional invasive autopsy.
- The international terminology suggested is post-mortem computed tomography (PMCT) and post-mortem magnetic resonance (PMMR).
- PMCT is used to identify single or multiple fatalities, either locally or using teleradiology.
- PMCT cannot be used to determine where a person died.
- The use of PMCT to consider a possible post-mortem interval is in its infancy. A number of time dependent changes can be observed on PMCT which should not be mistaken as antemortem pathology. Some may arise as a consequence of cardiopulmonary resuscitation.
- PMCT can be used as an adjunct to enhance a limited or full invasive autopsy or, under the correct circumstances, as a replacement to the invasive autopsy to consider how someone came by their death.
- To visualise the coronary arteries, an enhanced scan involving one of the published methods of PMCT angiography is required.
- Ventilated PMCT appears to assist in the consideration of lung pathology.
- Additional laboratory tests can be undertaken prior to or after enhanced PMCT (test dependent).

REFERENCES

1. Rutty GN. Are autopsies necessary? The role of computed tomography as a possible alternative to invasive autopsies. Rechtsmedizin 2007; 17:21–28.
2. Rutty G, Rutty J. Perceptions of near virtual autopsies. J Forensic Leg Med 2011; 18:306–309.
3. Rutty J, Morgan B, Rutty GN. Managing transformational change: implementing cross-sectional imaging into death investigation services in the United Kingdom. J Forensic Radiol Imaging 2014; 3:57-60
4. Jeffery A, Morgan B, Raj V, et al. The Criminal Justice System's considerations of so-called 'Near virtual Autopsies'; the East Midlands Experience. J Clin Path 2011; 64:711–717.
5. Rutty GN, Brogdon G, Dedouit F, et al. Terminology used in publications for post-mortem cross-sectional imaging. Int J Legal Med 2013; 127:465–466.
6. Eckert WG, Garland N. The history of the forensic application in radiology. Am J Forensic Med Pathol 1984; 5:53–56.
7. Wullenweber R, Shneider V, Grummer TH. A computer-tomographical examination of cranial bullet wounds (author's translation). Z Rechtsmedizin 1977; 80:227–246.
8. Kranz P, Holtas S. Postmortem computed tomography in a diving fatality. J Comput Assist Tomogr 1983; 7:132–134.
9. Donchin Y, Rivkind AI, Bar-Ziv J, et al. Utility of postmortem computed tomography in trauma victims. J Trauma 1994; 37:552–555.

10. Brookes JA, Hall-Craggs MA, Sams VR, et al. Non-invasive perinatal necropsy by magnetic resonance imaging. Lancet 1996; 348:1139–1141.
11. Thali MJ, Yen K, Schweitzer W, et al. Virtopsy, a new imaging horizon in forensic pathology: virtual autopsy by postmortem multislice computed tomography (MSCT) and magnetic resonance imaging (MRI) – a feasibility study. J Forensic Sci 2003; 48:386–403.
12. Baglivo M, Winklhofer S, Hatch GM, et al. The rise of forensic and post-mortem radiology – analysis of the literature between the year 2000 and 2011. J Forensic Radiol Imaging 2012; 1:3–9.
13. Rutty GN, Morgan B, O'Donnell C, et al. Forensic institutes across the world place CT or MRI scanners or both into their mortuaries. J Trauma 2008; 65:493–494.
14. Morgan B, Alminyah A, Carr A, et al. Use of post-mortem computed tomography in Disaster Victim Identification. Positional statement of the members of the Disaster Victim Identification working group of the International Society of Forensic Radiology and Imaging. JoFRI 2014; 2:114–116.
15. NHS Implementation Sub-Group of the Department of Health Post Mortem, Forensic and Disaster Imaging Group. Can cross-sectional imaging as an adjunct and/or alternative to the invasive autopsy be implemented within the NHS? , London, NHS. October 2012.
16. Culbert WC and Law FM. Identification by comparison of roentgenograms of nasal accessory sinuses and mastoid process. J Am Med Assoc 1927; 88:1634–1636.
17. Elliot R. The value of roentgenology in the identification of mutilated and burnt bodies. J Criminal Law Criminology 1953; 43:681–684.
18. Hayakawa M, Yamamoto S, Motani H, et al. Does imaging technology overcome problems of conventional post-mortem examination? A trial of computed tomography imaging for postmortem examination. Int J Legal Med 2006; 120:24–26.
19. Rutty GN, Robinson CE, BouHaidar R, et al. The role of mobile computed tomography in mass fatality incidents. J Forensic Sci 2007; 52:1343–1349.
20. Rutty GN, Robinson C, Morgan B, et al. Fimag: the United Kingdom disaster victim/forensic identification imaging system. J Forensic Sci 2009; 54:1438–1442.
21. Sidler M, Jackowski C, Dirnhofer R, et al. Use of multislice computed tomography in disaster victim identification advantages and limitations. Forensic Sci Int 2007; 169:118–128.
22. Martinez RM, Ptacek W, Schweitzer W, et al. CT-guided, minimally invasive, postmortem needle biopsy using the B-Rob II needle-positioning robot. J Forensic Sci 2014; 59:517–521.
23. O'Donnell C, Iino M, Mansharan K, Leditscke J, Woodford N. Contribution of postmortem multidetector CT scanning to identification of the deceased in a mass disaster: Experience gained from the 2009 Victorian bushfires. Forensic Sci Int. 2011; 205:15-28
24. Rutty GN, Alminyah A, Calla A, et al. Disaster Victim Identification. Positional statement of the members of the Disaster Victim Identification working group of the International Society of Forensic Radiology and Imaging; May 2013. J Forensic Radiol Imaging 2013; 1:218.
25. Morgan B, Alminyah A, Carr A, et al. Use of post-mortem computed tomography in Disaster Victim Identification. Positional statement of the members of the Disaster Victim Identification working group of the International Society of Forensic Radiology and Imaging. JoFRI 2014; 2:114–116.
26. Brough AL, Rutty GN, Black S, et al. Post-mortem computed tomography and 3D imaging: anthropological applications for juvenile remains. Forensic Sci Med Pathol 2012; 8:270–279.
27. Brough AL, Morgan B, Black S, et al. Post-mortem computed tomography age assessment of juvenile dentition: comparison against traditional OPT assessment. Int J Legal Med 2014; 128:653–658.
28. Brough AL, Morgan B, Robinson C, et al. A minimum data set approach to post-mortem computed tomography reporting for anthropological biological profiling. Forensic Sci Med Pathol 2014; 10:504–512.
29. Brough AL, Morgan B, Rutty GN. The basics of disaster victim identification. J Forensic Radiol Imaging 2015; 3:29–37.
30. Madea B (ed.). Estimation of the time since death, 3rd edn. London: CRC Press, 2015.
31. Shiotani S, Kohno M, Ohashi N, et al. Postmortem intravascular high-density fluid level (hypostasis): CT findings. J Comput Assist Tomogr 2002; 26:892–893.
32. Takahashi N, Satou C, Higuchi T, et al. Quantitative analysis of intracranial hypostasis: comparison of early postmortem and antemortem CT findings. Am J Roentgenol 2010; 195:W388–393.
33. Levy AD, Harke HT, Mallak CT. Postmortem imaging. MBCT features of post-mortem change and decomposition. Am J Forensic Med Pathol 2010; 31:12–17.
34. Jackowski C, Thali M, Aghayev E, et al. Postmortem imaging of blood and its characteristics using MSCT and MRI. Int J Legal Med 2006; 120:233–240.

35. Shiotani S, Kohno M, Ohashi N, et al. Hyperattenuating aortic wall on postmortem computed tomography (PMCT). Radiat Med 2002; 20:201–206.
36. Takahashi N, Higuchi T, Hirose Y, et al. Changes in aortic shape and diameters after death: comparison of early postmortem computed tomography with antemortem computed tomography. Forensic Sci Int 2013; 225:27–31.
37. Ishikawa N, Nishida A, Miyamori D, et al. Estimation of postmortem time based on aorta narrowing in CT imaging. J Forensic Leg Med 2013; 20:1075–1077.
38. Shiotani S, Kohno M, Ohashi N, et al. Postmortem computed tomographic (PMCT) demonstration of the relation between gastrointestinal (GI) distension and hepatic portal venous gas (HPVG). Radiat Med 2004; 22:25–29.
39. Asamura H, Ito M, Takayanagi K, et al. Hepatic portal venous gas on postmortem CT scan. Leg Med (Tokyo) 2005; 7:326–330.
40. Yamazaki K, Shiotani S, Ohashi N, et al. Hepatic portal venous gas and hyper-dense aortic wall as postmortem computed tomography finding. Leg Med (Tokyo) 2003; 5 Suppl 1:S338–341.
41. Yokota H, Yamamoto S, Horikoshi T, et al. What is the origin of intravascular gas on postmortem computed tomography? Leg Med (Tokyo) 2009; 11 Suppl 1:S252–255.
42. Egger C, Bize P, Vaucher P, et al. Distribution of artifactual gas on post-mortem multidetector computed tomography (MDCT). Int J Legal Med 2012; 126:3–12.
43. Singh MK, O'Donnell C, Woodford NW. Progressive gas formation in a deceased person during mortuary storage demonstrated on computed tomography. Forensic Sci Med Pathol 2009; 5:236–242.
44. Ishida M, Gonoi W, Hagiwara K, et al. Postmortem changes of the thyroid on computed tomography. Legal Med 2011; 13:318–322.
45. Bavat AR, Koopmarschap D, Klein WM. Postmortem interval: value of post-mortem cerebral CT. J Forensic Radiol Imaging 2014; 2:98 abstract 1.10.
46. Jeffery A, Morgan B, Raj V, et al. The Criminal Justice System's considerations of so-called 'Near virtual Autopsies'; the East Midlands Experience. J Clin Path 2011; 64:711–717.
47. Fryer EP, Traill ZC, Benamore RE, et al. High risk medicolegal autopsies: is a full postmortem examination necessary? J Clin Pathol 2013; 66:1–7.
48. Clarke M, McGregor A, Robinson C, et al. Identifying the correct cause of death: The role of post-mortem computed tomography in sudden unexplained death. J Forensic Radiol Imaging 2014; 2:210–212.
49. Flach PM, Egli TC, Bolliger SA, et al. 'Blind spots' in forensic autopsy: improved detection of retrobulbar hemorrhage and orbital lesions by postmortem computed tomography (PMCT). Legal Med 2016; 16:274–284.
50. Saunders S, Kotecha D, Morgan B, et al. Demonstrating the origin of cardiac air embolism using post-mortem computed tomography; an illustrated case. Leg Med (Tokyo) 2010; 13:79–82.
51. Maskell G and Wells M. RCR/RCPath statement on standards for medico-legal post-mortem cross-sectional imaging in adults. London: The Royal College of Radiologists and the Royal College of Pathologists. 2012.
52. Roberts IS, Benamore RE, Benbow EW, et al. Post-mortem imaging as an alternative to autopsy in the diagnosis of adult deaths: a validation study. Lancet 2012; 379:136–142.
53. Rutty GN, Duerden RM, Carter N, et al. Are coroner's autopsies necessary? A prospective study examining whether a 'view and grant' system of death certification could be introduced into England and Wales. J Clin Path 2001; 54:279–284.
54. Biggs MJP, Brown LJR, Rutty GN. Can cause of death be predicted from the pre-necropsy information provided in Coroners' cases? J Clin Path 2008; 61:124–126.
55. Morgan B, Sakamoto N, Shiotani S, et al. Postmortem computed tomography (PMCT) scanning with angiography (PMCTA): a description of three distinct methods. In: Rutty GN (ed). Essential of autopsy practice, advances, updates and emerging technologies. London: Springer, 2014:1–22.
56. Morgan B, Biggs MJ, Barber J, et al. Accuracy of targeted post-mortem computed tomography coronary angiography compared to assessment of serial histological sections. Int J Legal Med 2013; 127:809–817.
57. Adlam D, Joseph S, Robinson C, et al. Coronary optical coherence tomography: minimally invasive virtual histology as part of targeted post-mortem computed tomography angiography. Int J Leg Med 2013; 127:991–996.
58. Jackowski C, Sonnenschein M, Thali MJ, et al. Virtopsy: postmortem minimally invasive angiography using cross section techniques – implementation and preliminary results. J Forensic Sci 2005; 50:1175–1186.
59. Jackowski C, Bolliger S, Aghayev E, et al. Reduction of postmortem angiography-induced tissue edema by using polyethylene glycol as a contrast agent dissolver. J Forensic Sci 2006; 51:1134–1137.

60. Grabherr S, Doenz F, Steger B, et al. Multi-phase post-mortem CT angiography: development of a standardized protocol. Int J Legal Med 2011; 125:791–802.
61. Saunders SL, Morgan B, Raj V, et al. Targeted post-mortem computed tomography cardiac angiography: proof of concept. Int J Legal Med 2011; 125:609–616.
62. Roberts IS, Benamore RE, Peebles C, et al. Diagnosis of coronary artery disease using minimally invasive autopsy: evaluation of a novel method of post-mortem coronary CT angiography. Clin Radiol 2011; 66:645–650.
63. Robinson C, Barber J, Amoroso J, et al. Pump injector system applied to targeted post-mortem coronary artery angiography. Int J Legal Med 2012; 127:661–666.
64. Sakamoto N, Senoo S, Kamimura Y, et al. Case report: cardiopulmonary arrest on arrival case which underwent contrast-enhanced postmortem CT. JAAM 2009; 30:114–115.
65. Iizuka K, Sakamoto N, Kawasaki H, et al. Usefulness of contrast-enhanced postmortem CT. Innervision 2009; 24:89–92.
66. Zaporozhan J, Ley S, Eberhardt R, et al. Paired inspiratory/expiratory volumetric thin-slice CT scan for emphysema analysis – comparison of different quantitative evaluations and pulmonary function test. Chest 2005; 128:3212–3220.
67. Prosch H, Schaefer-Prokop CM, Eisenhuber E, et al. CT protocols in interstitial lung diseases – a survey among members of the European Society of Thoracic Imaging and a review of the literature. Eur Radiol 2013; 23:1553–1563.
68. Christe A, Flach P, Ross S, et al. Clinical radiology and postmortem imaging (Virtopsy) are not the same: Specific and unspecific postmortem signs. Legal Med 2010; 12:215–222.
69. Germerott T, Preiss US, Ebert LC, et al. A new approach in virtopsy: postmortem ventilation in multislice computed tomography. Leg Med (Tokyo) 2010; 12:276–279.
70. Grichnik KP, Shaw A. Update on one-lung ventilation: the use of continuous positive airway pressure ventilation and positive end-expiratory pressure ventilation – clinical application. Curr Opin Anaesthesiol 2009; 22:23–30 [Review].
71. Dreyfuss D, Saumon G. Ventilator-induced lung injury: lessons from experimental studies. Am J Respir Crit Care Med 1998; 157:294–323.
72. Germerott T, Flach PM, Preiss US, et al. Postmortem ventilation: a new method for improved detection of pulmonary pathologies in forensic imaging. Leg Med (Tokyo) 2012; 14:223–228.
73. Germerott T, Preiss US, Ross SG, et al. Postmortem ventilation in cases of penetrating gunshot and stab wounds to the chest. Leg Med (Tokyo) 2013; 15:298–302.
74. Robinson C, Biggs MJ, Amoroso J, et al. Post-mortem computed tomography ventilation; simulating breath holding. Int J Legal Med 2014; 128:139–146.
75. Rutty GN, Biggs MJ, Brough A, et al. Ventilated post-mortem computed tomography through the use of a definitive airway. Int J Legal Med 2015; 129:325-34.
76. Fronczek J, Hollingbury F, Biggs M, et al. The role of histology in forensic autopsies: is histological examination always necessary to determine a cause of death? Forensic Sci Med Pathol 2014; 10:39–43.
77. de la Grandmaison GL, Charlier P, Durigon M. Usefulness of systematic histological examination in routine forensic autopsy. J Forensic Sci 2010; 55:85–88.
78. Chatelain D, Hebert A, Trouillet N, et al. Effectiveness of histopathologic examination in a series of 400 forensic autopsies. [Article in French] Ann Pathol 2012; 32:4–13.
79. Molina DK, Wood LE, Frost RE. Is routine histopathologic examination beneficial in all medicolegal autopsies? Am J Forensic Med Pathol 2007; 28:1–3.
80. De-Giorgio F, Vetrugno G. Is histological examination always necessary to determine a cause of death? Of course it is! Forensic Sci Med Pathol 2014; 10:477–478.
81. Uchiyama T, Kakizaki E, Kozawa S, et al. A new molecular approach to help conclude drowning as a cause of death: simultaneous detection of eight bacterioplankton species using real-time PCR assays with TaqMan probes. Forensic Sci Int 2012; 222:11–26.
82. Terry R. Needle necropsy. J Clin Pathol 1955; 8:38–41.
83. Aghayev E, Thali MJ, Sonnenschein M, et al. Post-mortem tissue sampling using computed tomography guidance. Forensic Sci Int 2007; 166:199–203.
84. Aghayev E, Ebert LC, Christe A, et al. CT data-based navigation for post-mortem biopsy – a feasibility study. J Forensic Leg Med 2008; 15:382–387.
85. Ebert LC, Ptacek W, Naether S, et al. Virtobot – a multi-functional robotic system for 3D surface scanning and automatic post mortem biopsy. Int J Med Robot 2010; 6:18–27.

86. Martinez RM, Ptacek W, Schweitzer W, et al. CT-guided, minimally invasive, postmortem needle biopsy using the B-Rob II needle-positioning robot. J Forensic Sci 2014; 59:517–521.

87. Ebert LC, Ptacek W, Breitbeck R, et al. Virtobot 2.0: the future of automated surface documentation and CT-guided needle placement in forensic medicine. Forensic Sci Med Pathol 2014; 10:179–186.

88. Ebert LC, Ptacek W, Fürst M, et al. Minimally invasive postmortem telebiopsy. J Forensic Sci 2012; 57:528–530.

89. Rutty GN, Barber J, Amoroso J, et al. The effect on cadaver blood DNA identification by the use of targeted and whole body post-mortem computed tomography angiography. Forensic Sci Med Pathol 2013; 9:489–495.

90. Rutty GN, Smith P, Visser T, et al. The effect on toxicology, biochemistry and immunology investigations by the use of targeted post-mortem computed tomography angiography. Forensic Sci Int 2013; 225:42–47.

91. Grabherr S, Widmer C, Iglesias K, et al. Postmortem biochemistry performed on vitreous humor after postmortem CT-angiography. Leg Med (Tokyo) 2012; 14:297–303.

92. Palmiere C, Grabherr S, Augsburger M. Postmortem computed tomography angiography, contrast medium administration and toxicological analyses in urine. Leg Med (Tokyo) 2014:S1344–6223(14)00176-X.

93. Palmiere C, Egger C, Grabherr S, et al. Postmortem angiography using femoral cannulation and postmortem microbiology. Int J Legal Med 2015; 129:861–867.

Chapter 6

Review of postgraduate medical education in the UK

Davinder PS Sandhu

INTRODUCTION

Postgraduate medical education (PGME) is defined as that phase of medical education in which doctors develop competencies after completion of their basic medical qualification. This has to be achieved under a proper governance framework of selection, curriculum delivery, educational supervision, formative and summative feedback including postgraduate examinations and credentialing. Postgraduate training in histopathology is unique as it is a complex specialty consisting of many separate disciplines, each of which require detailed knowledge of the disease process and diagnostic skills. Such training has to be within a proper governance structure to produce a fit-for-purpose 21st century pathologist who is familiar other facets such as genetics and the genome project, immunological testing of tissue as well as radiological investigations. Details of postgraduate training in histopathology are discussed at the end of the chapter after an overview of the development of postgraduate training in the UK.

In the UK postgraduate training occurs under the auspices of the Deaneries [1] (now called PGME offices in England) and the General Medical Council (GMC) which is the UK regulating body accountable to Parliament.

In England the PGME offices are part of the Local Education and Training Boards (LETBs). LETBs are regional offices of Health Education England with a Director of Education and Quality who is the responsible officer for multi-professional education and can be a Postgraduate Medical Dean or from other allied health professionals.

In UK medicine, PGME involves several stages:
- Preregistration year 1 as part of the 2-year Foundation Programme (FP)
- Completion of second Foundation year with achievement of foundation competencies. This is the first stage of postgraduate training
- Core training (CT)
- Higher specialist training
- Credentialing
- Continuous professional development

Davinder PS Sandhu MD, FRCS (Ed Urol), FRCS (Eng & Glas), CertMedEd, FRCPE, FDSRCS (Eng), FRCGP(Hons) FHEA, Medical University Bahrain, Adliya, Bahrain. Email: dsandhu@rcsi-mub.com (for correspondence)

GMC REGISTRATION

Foundation year 1 (FY1) allows students to undertake their training with provisional registration from the GMC. Successful completion of FY1 leads to full registration. No trainee can undertake PGME unless they have full registration with the GMC. The preparation and process of PGME start within the continuum of the undergraduate course. For example, final year medical students in the UK undertake a national drug prescribing examination that is conducted by the Medical Schools Council. They also undertake preparation for professional practice that gives experience of working in the acute specialties, taking on additional responsibilities and shadowing an FY1 doctor.

EVOLUTION OF PGME IN THE UK

PGME is a dynamic and an iterative process that evolves over many decades. To understand the current structure of UK PGME, there needs to be an appreciation of important milestones that have contributed to its development. The key reports are:

- The Calman report
- Modernising medical careers (MMCs)
- The Tooke report on modernising medical careers
- The Collins report on foundation training
- The Temple report on the impact of the European Working Time Regulation
- The shape of training

The Calman report

Prior to the Calman Report in 1993 'Hospital doctors, training for the future' [2], PGME in the UK was a time-based apprenticeship and not competency-based. The basic structure after medical school was a preregistration year as House Officer (FY1), followed by CT as Senior House Officer (SHO), then competitively into Registrar and then Senior Registrar positions that would, if successful, lead to a Consultant post. A Consultant position was not guaranteed. In the competitive specialties, it was not uncommon for trainees to labour several years in each of the grades until being able to move onto the next tier, and being appointed as Consultant in their early forties or later. There was no formal system such as a certification of completion of training that recognised that training to the level of a year 1 Consultant had been achieved. The value of primary care was also diminished by a hierarchal attitude that if you were unsuccessful in hospital practice, you could always become a General Practitioner (GP). In addition, the European Commission criticised the UK for infringing its directive on specialist recognition. These deficiencies encouraged the then Chief Medical Officer Professor Kenneth Calman to address PGME and meet the European Directive [2].

The report recommended a certificate of completion of specialist training (CCST) with a curriculum for each specialty, structured training programmes that combined the registrar and senior registrar grades to ensure continuity, progression through training based on formal annual assessments of competence and much shorter training in most specialties. The Calman Report [3] confirmed that the Medical Royal Colleges and Postgraduate Deans would contribute to the planning and delivery of the new structure and curriculum. Crucially, this was not a 'Big Bang' approach but the new specialist training was to start for general surgery and clinical radiology first in December 1995, and for all other specialties between April 1996 and April 1997. This staged implementation was essential as the complexity in medicine with approximately 60 specialties, each with its own curriculum and delivery difficulties, was enormous.

All eligible trainees were allocated a national training number (NTN) by their Deanery. Overseas doctors, defined as those who were not nationals of countries in the European Economic Area, were also able to transfer, depending on their rights of residency or available permitted time for postgraduate training in Britain. A new innovative programme was created called fixed-term training appointment (FTTA) that did not have an NTN, but was equivalent to an NTN programme and could count towards a CCST if subsequently appointed to a post with a designated NTN. These FTTA appointments were useful to fill gaps in specialist registrar programmes replacing the often unplanned and unstructured 'locum' appointments [3].

The CCST was a definite educational end point, and enabled entry on the medical register with specialist recognition equivalent to other European countries. The training progression would ensure that the content of the curriculum was clearly defined and progress monitored through yearly educational appraisal, confirming the trainee's competence and skill. The Royal Colleges were tasked with providing detailed descriptions of standards and methods of assessment. Furthermore these were made available to both assessors and trainees for transparency, and the outcome of reviews of progress monitored by Colleges, and a summary record kept in the training file by the Postgraduate Dean.

There was also the recommendation that the period of training including core (SHO) should not exceed 7 years after full registration for most specialties. This latter goal has still not been achieved though this initiative did enhance many aspects of training such as assessment and feedback.

There was a new application process and new standards for shortlisting applicants, obtaining references, and convening appointment panels. Thus, there was improvement in objectivity and fairness in appointments.

An aspect new to many was the introduction of training agreements between the trainee, postgraduate Dean, and the hospitals where training was to take place. There was an expectation of commitment by Consultants, to be regular in service tuition, and protected time for trainees to study and be trained with a reciprocal commitment from the trainee to engage with the training.

Configuring higher specialist training was a massive undertaking, and not surprisingly at that stage little attention was given to SHO training who became known as the lost tribe.

To address the deficiencies of preregistration and SHO training and create a streamlined programme linking preregistration and core with higher specialist training, the MMC initiative was created in 2002 [5].

Modernising medical careers

The rationale for MMC arose from the problems affecting the SHO grade summarised in the document 'Unfinished Business, 2002'[5] written by the then Chief Medical Officer for England Sir Liam Donaldson, but there were also three other areas that needed to be addressed:

- Create an educational and career pathway for Staff Grade and Associate Specialist (SAS) doctors.
- Supersede the preregistration year with a 2-year FP that would need a curriculum and an operational framework.
- Need to comply with the European Working Time Directive (EWTD) regulations.

SHO grade

The SHOs lacked a defined career structure, leaving many of them in short-term posts that lasted only 6 months and not in a formal training programme. This meant that there was no defined end point or time limit to SHO training. Some trainees unable to progress were left in this grade for 10 years or more and hence the lost tribe. These trainees were poorly supervised with limited career advice and there were no defined competencies to meet the requirements for training.

'Unfinished Business' set out key principles for the SHO grade: training should be programme-based, time-limited, broad-based to begin with, flexible and tailored to individual needs.

Foundation programme

To achieve the reform of the SHO grade, it was proposed to create a 2-year FP [5] that would then seamlessly lead to run-through training consisting of basic specialist and higher specialist training. Foundation would mainly comprise six 4-month posts including General Practice. Progression through the programme would be subject to satisfactory performance and assessments. Every Deanery created a 2-year coupled FP for the medical students.

An advantage of foundation was that it gave young trainees opportunities to experience a variety of specialties. There was encouragement to create 5% of posts in shortage specialties and also to develop academic programmes.

SAS doctors

In July 2003, less than a year after 'Unfinished Business', the Department of Health (DH) published another Consultation paper, 'Choice and Opportunity' [6]. This paper addressed the difficulties SAS doctors were facing. The SAS doctors were outside the formal training system and without consultant or GP status. The SAS doctors, also known as Nonconsultant Career Grade doctors, had several disadvantages:

- There was a lack of a recognised career structure for the 12,500 SAS doctors.
- The type of work undertaken lacked variation and tended to be routine and monotonous with little training or professional development.

MMC established principles for reforming the careers of SAS doctors. Namely:

- There should be clear criteria for doctors entering SAS posts including the possibility of career progression through the acquisition of recognised competencies.
- Doctors in SAS posts should have access to training, continuous professional development and careers advice.

This reinforces the fact that PGME and training is not cocooned. It is dependent on the reforms and aspirations of DH. Because PGME is experiential learning and based in the patient environment, it is affected by what is happening to the NHS structure and finances.

The other pressures in the NHS at that time were:

- Widespread deficits across the NHS in 2004–2005, putting pressure on all NHS organisations to reduce expenditure, making educational budgets vulnerable.
- Structural reorganisation and reduction in number of SHAs and Primary Care Trusts (PCTs) taking place in 2006, creating further uncertainty and distraction for NHS organisations during the planning and implementation of the MMC reforms.
- Implementation of the EWTD reforms, restricting junior doctors to a maximum of 58 hours per week by 2004, with a further reduction to 48 hours by 2009. This meant that the NHS could not rely on junior doctors working long hours to prop up the service.

- The NHS Plan (2000) [7] set out a commitment to a health service increasingly delivered by fully trained doctors rather than those in training. This created pressure to reduce the minimum training times for completion of specialist training and the service contribution by trainees. The NHS Plan also promised to increase the self sufficiency of the NHS workforce, underpinned by a major expansion in undergraduate student numbers, a process that had begun in 1997. Medical school student numbers rose by around 60% between 1999 and 2005; four new medical schools were created as part of this expansion.
- In 2003, a new regulator for postgraduate medical training, the PGME and Training Board (PMETB) was created [8]. This was in part of a general move away from a self-regulated medical profession in light of high profile failings, such as unreported excess deaths in paediatric cardiac surgery at Bristol Royal Infirmary [9] and unconsented storage of pathological specimens at Alder Hey [10].

Crucially, 'The Next Steps paper' in 2004 [11] signalled the intention to adopt 'a single, run-through approach' for the delivery of specialist, including GP, training programmes. The paper clearly set out that Specialist Programmes and General Practice would be developed to provide a seamless training process that would see all those emerging from FPs entering a training programme leading directly to the award of a Certificate of Completion of Training (CCT). Entry will be competitive but, subject to satisfactory progress, no further competition would be needed before the completion of training (**Figure 6.1**).

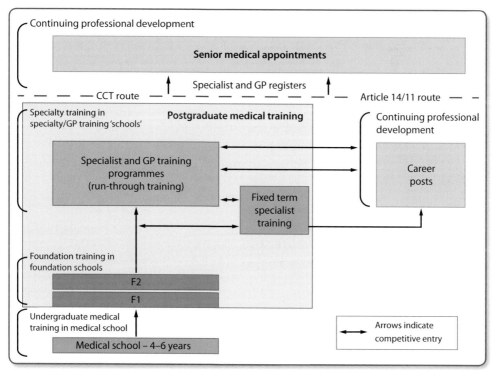

Figure 6.1 Structure of training proposed by Modernising Medical Careers team. With permission from Department of Health, Modernising Medical Careers team, November 2005.

The failings of MMC [12]

These are important lessons for all those involved in PGME. Although the aspirations of MMC as outlined above were supported, the implementation created a massive loss of confidence in the system and delivery of MMC. More specifically, the areas of concern were:

- This was a 'Big Bang' approach with no pilots of any speciality and subsequent assessment of outcome.
- The complexity of dealing with creating a run-through programme, a high stakes decision, particularly in the competitive specialties, where there was already a large cohort of trainees in the system who had committed to the speciality was not appreciated. If experienced trainees were to be appointed then this went against the grain of entry into run-through from Foundation. If inexperienced Foundation trainees were appointed with no recognition of research, academic achievements and competencies of senior trainees then this seemed unfair. In the end to support Foundation trainees, experience and examination performance were not part of the explicit selection criteria.
- There was unsubstantiated belief that previous systems of selection into specialist training had been riven with patronage and therefore a computerised centralised admission system, Medical Training Application Service (MTAS) was chosen for recruitment into Specialist Training Year 1. As a result, some apparently high quality candidates were not selected. The interview panels also had little training and lacked confidence in negotiating the new system.
- Trainees were concerned about missing out on entry into a programme and therefore to hedge their bets, made multiple applications. This caused a huge system overload, with failure of MTAS to negotiate over 100,000 applications. The confidentiality of application data was eroded in some instances and some trainees' application process stalled.
- There were concerns about forced prematurity of choice of final speciality and perceived rigidity and failure of more ad hoc training opportunities.

These were just some of the concerns that among a huge educational and political angst led to the Tooke Review 'Aspiring to Excellence' [12]. There was a call not only to address PGME but the wider issues of how health policy is developed, workforce planning, the role of the doctor, career development and regulation of doctors and medical education.

Aspiring to excellence – the Tooke review [12]

This was the first of many reviews that progressed PGME and some of the conclusions of the inquiry were:

1. MMC failed to address the role of doctors at the various stages of their careers. Urgent attention should be given to linking PGME with workforce planning.
2. PMETB should be merged with the GMC to facilitate economies of scale.
3. The structure of postgraduate training should be modified to provide a broad-based platform and for some competitive specialties, core should be decoupled from higher specialist training.
4. The creation of a new body called Medical Education England (MEE). This would host the ring fenced education budget, and relate to the medical workforce advisory machinery and act as the professional interface between policy development and implementation on matters relating to PGME.

5. The FP should be uncoupled for CT and a 3-year CT comprising of FY2/CT1/CT2 should be created.
6. Concerns were raised about the EWTD.

Time for training: a review of the impact of the EWTD on the quality of training [13]

One of the concerns of the profession supported by the Tooke inquiry was the impact of the EWTD and later when in law the EWTD on PGME. The reduction in working hours to 48 per week in August 2009 was having a detrimental effect in the craft specialties. There was a conflict for the NHS between delivering safe service for its patients and high quality training. Temple concluded that the experiential model of learning had to change dramatically if the NHS was to continue to produce well-trained and safe professionals. His motto became 'make every moment count' [13]. Some of the key recommendations are:

- Trainers and trainees must use the learning opportunities in every clinical situation.
- Handovers can be an effective learning experience when supervised by senior staff.
- The coordinated, integrated use of simulation and technology can provide a safe, controlled environment and accelerate learning.
- Mentoring and support for trainees must be improved.
- Trainees must be involved in the decision-making and implementation of training innovations that affect their present and future careers.
- Services must be designed and configured to deliver high quality patient care and training.
- As the ratio of trainees to consultants changes, it may no longer be feasible to train in all hospitals.
- Rotas require organisation and effective management to maximise training in 48 hours.
- Multidisciplinary team-working must be used to support training.
- Consultants must work flexibly and be more directly responsible for the delivery of 24/7 and out of hours care.
- The EWTD leads to an improved work life balance. Enhanced supervision of trainees out of hours leads to safer patient care and reduces the loss of daytime training opportunities.

Thus in the NHS, a trainee needs to learn in a service-based environment and the learning opportunity in every clinical situation must be realised.

Foundation for excellence: an evaluation of the FP [14]

While Temple addressed the issues about the EWTD [13], some trainers and trainees particularly in surgical specialties had undervalued the second FY and therefore in its conclusion, the Tooke report recommended the decoupling of the 2-year programme and making FY2 part of CT. Many in education and particularly those in charge of developing the FP, considered this to be a retrograde step. In order to address this issue, MEE requested a review of Foundation especially as 5 years had passed since its introduction in 2005. The Collins' report [14] concluded that the FP had many strengths, but there were questions over key aspects of design, content, safety and quality. The principle recommendations were to prioritise patient safety, the interests of the trainees and the need to improve quality and efficiency in a transparent way. Crucially it did not recommend decoupling of the FP but deferred this for further 5 years till 2015 when longer term benefit, strength and weaknesses could be evaluated. At present, the FP remains a 2-year coupled programme.

Both of these reports had the common theme of better use of the expanded consultant workforce and concerns that some of the junior trainees are asked to practice beyond their level of competence, and without appropriate or adequate supervision.

'Shape of Training' [15]

The next and most recent major review of PGME was 'Shape of Training' in 2013 led by Professor David Greenaway under the aegis of a four-country (England, Scotland, Wales and Northern Ireland) sponsorship board, including the Academy of Medical Royal Colleges, Council of Postgraduate Medical Deans, Medical Schools Council and the GMC. The drivers for this review were the change in population demographics such as an aging population with multiple comorbidities, more demand for care in the community, pressures on dealing with mental health, increasing demand for primary care and urgent care in emergency departments, together with the feminisation of the medical workforce and the resulting impact on work life balance. Within a specialty there is considerable super-specialisation with the difficulty of not having sufficient generalists who can staff emergency rotas. Additional pressure is created by health inequalities and increasing patient expectations.

The key recommendations of the report are:
- Patients and the public need more doctors who are capable of delivering safe and effective general care in broad specialties across a range of different settings.
- There will remain a need to train some highly specialised doctors to meet local patient and workforce needs.
- Medicine has to be a sustainable career with opportunities for doctors to change roles and specialties throughout their careers.
- Local workforce and patient needs should drive opportunities to train in new specialties or to credential in specific areas.
- Doctors in academic training pathways need a training structure that is flexible enough to allow them to move in and out of clinical training, while meeting the competencies and standards of that training.
- Full registration should move from end of FY1 to the point of graduation from medical school, providing the graduates are fit for purpose in that role. This is probably the most radical of all the recommendations.
- Implementation of the recommendations must be UK-wide and a delivery group should be formed to oversee the implementation of the recommendations.

Greenway supports the FP but emphasises that throughout medical school and Foundation, doctors must have opportunities to support and follow patients through their entire care pathway. After completion of the FP, all trainees will enter broad-based speciality training. Specialties or areas of practice will be grouped together. These groupings will be characterised by patient care themes such as women's health, child health and mental health. To achieve this, there will need to be common clinical objectives set out in the speciality curricula approved by the GMC. Such broad-based speciality training will last between 4 years and 6 years depending on the speciality requirements. The exit point of PGME will be the Certificate of Speciality Training (CST). It marks the point at which doctors are able to practice independently in their identified scope of practice while working in multiprofessional teams. All CST holders should be part of the emergency on call rotas.

Across all specialities, training doctors should develop generic capabilities that reinforce professionalism in their medical practice.

An innovative recommendation is that during postgraduate training, doctors should be given opportunities to spend up to a year working in a related speciality or undertaking education, leadership or management work. This encompasses a broader opportunity from the current Out of Programme Experience that tends to be related to clinical training or research. This year can be taken at any time during training, and will allow the trainees to become more rounded professionals.

Flexibility is offered by giving doctors who want to change specialties, either within or between speciality groups, the provision to transfer relevant competencies they have acquired in one specialty to their new area of practice. This will include learning during the optional year and generic capabilities. By recognising previous learning and experiences, retraining in new areas should be shorter. More flexibility will also apply to clinical academic training pathways. Doctors on this pathway would be able to focus their academic training in their academic or research area while also undertaking broad-based training. Time spent in academic experiences will be counted within training, but if considerable time is undertaken for instance in doctoral research studies then the training time can be extended. In exceptional circumstances, doctors in clinical academic training may be able to restrict their clinical practice to special interest or subspecialty areas.

Post CST, some doctors will be able to specialise further by gaining additional expertise in particular interest areas and subspecialty training through formal and quality assured training programmes, leading to a credential in that area. These programmes will be driven by patient and workforce needs and may be commissioned by employers as well as other PGME organisations such as Higher Education Institutions (HEIs), Health Education England and Local Education and Training Boards.

Most doctors will work in the general area of their broad speciality, based on patient and workforce needs, throughout their careers. They will be expected to maintain and develop their skills in their speciality area, and their generic capabilities through continuing professional development to meet the requirements of revalidation. Learning through experience and reflection on their practice and patient outcomes will help give them the depth of knowledge and skills necessary to master their speciality area. Doctors will also have options at any point in their careers to develop their education, management and leadership roles (**Figure 6.2**).

Challenges with implementation of shape of training:

1. This chapter has already reinforced the iterative nature of the development of PGME and shape of training will be no exception. A four-nation steering group has been established to advise the government. Meanwhile the DH has asked HEE in its mandate [17] for a more detailed and fully costed work programme, including an impact assessment.

2. Registration at the point of graduation may not happen till 2021 as this will require an act of parliament and time for implementation. There is the opportunity to establish a national licensing examination that could also replace Professional and Linguistic Assessments Board examination for non-European doctors.

3. In CT, creating common curricula encompassing common objectives leading to themed programmes has good rationale, but will require a major undertaking from the Royal Colleges and the Academy of Royal Medical Colleges. This will need to include assessment of competence and progression across specialties as in broad-based training. There is the added advantage of ensuring transferable competencies.

4. Ensuring all postgraduate trainings to the level of CST within 4–6 years may create difficulties if trainees take a year out for their professional development. This maybe a

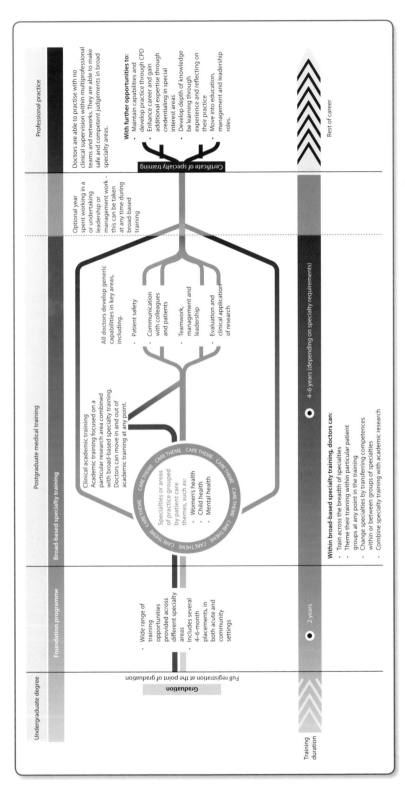

Figure 6.2 Shape of training – structure of postgraduate medical training. CPD, continuing professional development [15] © 2013 Shape of Training.

particular challenge for the craft specialties. However the Annual Review of Competence Progression should be able to address the need for additional time. CST holders will be consultants capable of independent practice and all will have to participate in emergency on-call rotas. It is important not to focus on the time but more on what knowledge, skills and attributes are needed to be a successful CST holder.

5. Every speciality will need some super specialised Consultants, and creation of credentialed post CST fellowships will be a huge undertaking. This could create difficulties, if employers and professional organisations were not able to access the appropriate level of investment and this could lead to a direct negative effect on patient care. It is anticipated that the majority of the funding will be a lift from the current funding within the CCT programme. Credentialing will also give opportunity for Consultants to develop later in their career.

Nevertheless, the strength of the Greenway report is that it has not ignored the difficult areas, and made a genuine attempt to come up with rich ideas for how to create a fit for purpose workforce that meets the needs of patients, and also shorten the medical training within a financially viable envelope.

INFLUENCE ON AND DEVELOPMENT OF HISTOPATHOLOGY TRAINING

Histopathology training consists of neuropathology, cytopathology, paediatric pathology and forensic pathology. As a specialty it has its own challenges in that there is an increasing range of specialist branches, and because it is an area in which diagnostic processes have great importance. To meet these challenges, the workforce must be recruited from the best of dedicated applicants. Prior to the immigration restriction the competition ration for histopathology was much higher, but in 2014 it was 1.8:1 [18].

Health Education England and the Royal College of Pathologists and its training committee have been developing novel structured training programmes in histopathology to improve the quality of applicants by making the programmes more structured and flexible with modular teaching, as with other specialties' national recruitment. Applicants must have completed the Foundation Programme within the last three years and must not have been in a previous histopathology training scheme. Recruitment is at ST1 level and the trainees are assigned to a local School of Histopathology.

Schools of Histopathology

As part of the NHS Plan and the NHS Cancer Plan, the Schools project was introduced by the NHS Modernisation committee in 2000 to respond to increasing demands for laboratory services, especially in cancer care. Their intention was to improve standards of teaching and train cohorts of trainees together more effectively in order to produce a greater number of trained histopathologists [19].

These schools started as a pilot and were initially based in Southampton, Leicester and Leeds. Since 2008, they have expanded to 16 throughout the United Kingdom. This approach was also developed for radiology. The advantage of the Schools structure was that the trainees obtained hands-on experience in their local Trusts but had 3 weeks of a structured national training programme over the course of the year. This has evolved into a week of national teaching, two weeks of regional teaching and a half day every fortnight in the regions. In 2005 there were 108 places but more recently the numbers are around 70 – 80 NTNs.

Aptitude assessment

This is unusual in specialty training. During the first year, normally at 9 months, the trainees are assessed and if they do not pass they are given one further assessment.

Modular training

The traditional training pathway takes 5 years. However, the trainees have to select a minimum of one module and a maximum of two from autopsy, research methodology and gynecology cytology. If they select two modules the training time is expanded to 5 and a half years [20].

Late entry at ST3

Those students who have a background in neurosciences or psychiatry can be recruited into ST3 during which they complete a year's general histopathology training, and then in ST4 – ST5, they continue to develop their expertise in neuropathology. A similar scheme exists for those with paediatric training wishing to enter paediatric pathology. After obtaining their FRCPath many trainees will opt to study in specialised units in areas such as uropathology and cardiovascular.

Curriculum development

Histopathology is currently receiving a high profile within the 100,000 Genome Project. All trainees will need a working knowledge of genetic influence on disease, chromosomal testing, mutations, and how chemotherapy and other treatment modalities need to be tailored to individual patients' genetic expression. The specialty has developed its resources of long distance learning and Masters programmes, particularly through links at individual school trainee websites.

Key points for clinical practice

- Postgraduate medical education is a lifelong vocation and has to be patient centred.
- A health organisation's workforce must be provided with the opportunity to develop the skills necessary to meet the needs of patients and the health service, and they should be consulted about future plans; in other words a 'bottom up' approach rather than 'top down'.
- Organisational development requires flexibility and preparing for the future. However, the impact of disruptive innovations should be appreciated, schemes piloted and 'big bang' approaches avoided.
- Constant structure change is expensive and can lead to loss of skilled staff.
- Medical schools should reassure patients and employers that their graduates are fit to practice.
- Medical students should receive regular career advice which provides them with a clear understanding of what can be expected in a medical career.
- The generic curricula for PGME should implement the GMC's 'Good Medical Practice' guidance and ensure that professional competencies, such as patient safety, dealing with uncertainty, communication skills, inter-professional team work and leadership, are implemented.

> • The development of the histopathology curriculum is an iterative process and therefore depends on close collaboration between Health Education England and the Royal College of Pathologists, not only in emerging specialist skills but also in workforce planning.

REFERENCES

1. Sandhu DPS. Deaneries: what do they do? BMJ Careers 2012; 3:1–4.
2. Department of Health. Hospital doctors: training for the future. The report of the working group on specialist medical training. London: HMSO, 1993.
3. Biggs J. New arrangements for specialist training in Britain. BMJ 1995; 311:1242–1243.
4. Donaldson L. Unfinished business: proposals for reform of the senior house officer grade – a paper for consultation. London: Department of Health, 2002.
5. Modernising Medical Careers. Operational framework for foundation training. London: The Stationary Office, 2005.
6. Choice and opportunity: modernising medical careers for non-consultant career grade doctors – summary of outcome. London: Department of Health, 2004.
7. The NHS plan: a plan for investment, a plan for reform. London: Department of Health, 2000.
8. Postgraduate Medical Education and Training: The Medical Education Standards Board, a paper for consultation. London: Department of Health, 2001.
9. The Bristol Royal infirmary inquiry final report. London: The Stationery Office, 2001.
10. The Royal Liverpool children's inquiry: summary and recommendations. London: HMSO, 2001.
11. The UK Health Departments. The next steps – the future shape of foundation, specialist and general practice training programmes. London: Department of Health, 2004.
12. John Tooke. Aspiring to Excellence. Findings and final recommendations of the Independent Inquiry into Modernising Medical Careers. London: Modernising Medical Careers Inquiry, 2008.
13. Temple J. Time for training. A Review of the impact of the European Working Time Directive on the quality of training. Leeds: Health Education England, 2010.
14. Collins J. Foundation for excellence. An evaluation of the Foundation Programme, Leeds: Medical Education England, 2010.
15. David Greenaway. Shape of training: securing the future of excellent patient care. Final report of the independent review. London: Shape of Training, 2013.
16. House of Commons Health Committee. Modernising medical careers: third report of session 2007–08 (vol. 1). London: The Stationery Office Limited, 2008.
17. Williams, L. Delivering high quality, effective, compassionate care: developing the right people with the right skills and the right values. London: Department of Health, 2013.
18. Kennedy C and Howes J. Specialty training applications for 2015: competition ratios and changes to the process. London: BMJ Careers. 2014.
19. Gallagher PJ, Dixon MF, Heard S, et al. An initiative to reform senior house officer training in histopathology. Br J Hosp Med 2003;64: 302–305.
20. Joint Committee on Pathology Training. Curriculum for specialty training in histopathology. The London: Royal College of Pathologists, 2010.

Chapter 7

Pathology of gestational trophoblastic disease

Neil James Sebire

INTRODUCTION

Gestational trophoblastic disease [GTD, also known as gestational trophoblastic neoplasia (GTN)] is a term used to describe a group of conditions, all of which are characterised by abnormal trophoblast proliferation. These are generally divided into the pregnancy-related premalignant conditions of hydatidiform mole and a separate group of gestational trophoblastic tumours (GTTs), although, of course, there is potential overlap between these conditions [1]. Because their clinical presentation, management and histological features are quite different, for the purposes of this review these groups of conditions will be addressed separately. It should be recognised that the main rationale for accurate identification of cases of hydatidiform mole is to ensure that they can be recognised, followed up and managed in order to prevent their later clinical presentation as overt GTTs.

In general, GTTs arise from any preceding pregnancy, but the risk of this occurring following normal pregnancy is around 1 in 50,000 compared with significantly higher risks following hydatidiform molar pregnancy. Following a complete hydatidiform mole (CHM), 15% of cases will require chemotherapy for persistent gestational trophoblastic disease (pGTD), and following a partial hydatidiform mole (PHM) the incidence is around 1 in 200 cases [2]. With the accurate identification of hydatidiform mole and subsequent maternal serum human chorionic gonadotropin (hCG) surveillance protocols, the vast majority of cases requiring chemotherapy are now based on the detection of plateauing or rising hCG concentrations in the absence of other clinical features and no tissue diagnosis. Therefore, pGTD is a generic group which may represent persistence of molar villi or invasive mole, whereas others may represent very early development of choriocarcinoma (CC). The term GTT is therefore reserved for those cases with a definite clinical- or tissue-based diagnosis of CC, placental site trophoblastic tumour (PSTT) or epithelioid trophoblastic tumour (ETT).

Regardless of other factors, cases of pGTD diagnosed on surveillance have essentially a 100% cure rate with first- or second-line chemotherapy. The vast majority of cases of CC are also cured with current chemotherapeutic regimes, although there remains associated rare mortality, usually with cases presenting late with advanced or complicated

Neil James Sebire MB BS BClinSci MD FRCOG FRCPath Professor of Pathology, Institute of Child Health/UCL; Consultant Pathologist, Trophoblastic Disease Unit, Department of Cancer Medicine, Charing Cross Hospital (Imperial Hospitals NHS Trust), Fulham Palace Road, London, UK. Email: n.sebire@ucl.ac.uk (for correspondence)

disease [3]. The prognosis for PSTT/ETT is largely dependent on histological staging and underlying biological factors. These require treatment with primary hysterectomy with the vast majority of stage 1 cases being cured and higher stage cases requiring adjuvant chemotherapy. For reasons that remain uncertain, PSTT/ETT has a significantly worse prognosis in cases occurring >48 months following the last known pregnancy regardless of other factors [4]. Finally, although rates of pGTD/CC are increased following hydatidiform mole, it should be recognised that GTT may develop from any conception, molar or nonmolar, in which placental tissue is present.

CLASSIFICATION OF GTD

The classification system provided here, and most commonly used, is based on the World Health Organization (WHO) classification of tumors [1], recognising the following entities.
- *Hydatidiform moles*: These are abnormal conceptions, all of which demonstrate dysmorphic placental chorionic villi and abnormal trophoblast proliferation. These are classified as CHMs or PHMs based on histological and/or genetic findings. Rare specific subtypes are now recognised, including familial biparental CHM and mosaic CHM. All hydatidiform moles have increased risk of subsequent development of pGTN (persistent gestational trophoblastic neoplasia)/GTT, hence the rationale for their accurate detection and subsequent hCG surveillance.
- *Gestational trophoblastic tumours:* These are malignant epithelial tumours in which the neoplastic component demonstrates phenotypes of villous trophoblast (choriocarcinoma), or nonvillous interstitial trophoblast (PSTT and ETT). GTTs are almost always in the absence of chorionic villi (intraplacental CC being the exception). Although slightly controversial, CC occurring coexistent with molar villi is not currently recognised as an entity by the WHO.

pGTN is not a histological subtype, but rather a generic term representing all cases of postmolar disease in which hCG concentrations are plateauing or rising, hence requiring chemotherapy. The vast majority of all cases requiring chemotherapy are now therefore identified biochemically with no other clinical features and without a tissue diagnosis being available. This, therefore, may represent persistence of molar villi, invasive mole or early development of CC, all of which are treated in the similar manner initially.

MANAGEMENT OVERVIEW

The main aim of early recognition of hydatidiform mole is to allow surveillance with hCG monitoring in order that persistent disease can be detected early and treated successfully with the minimum of chemotherapy [2,3]. Changes in contemporary obstetric practice have resulted in the majority of cases in the UK now being evacuated in the late first trimester. Specifically, the routine early pregnancy assessment ultrasound scans and ultrasound assessment are now used as the first-line investigation for women presenting with vaginal bleeding in pregnancy. Therefore, it is now exceedingly uncommon for hydatidiform moles to present with features such as an enlarged uterus and other changes secondary to advanced disease. By far the most frequent presentation now is either nonspecific vaginal bleeding followed by diagnosis of a failed pregnancy or incidental detection of miscarriage on routine ultrasound examination. It should be highlighted that the vast majority of hydatidiform moles that undergo ultrasound examination are not recognised as molar on scan (although those are more likely to be CHMs), the majority simply are diagnosed as 'missed miscarriage' or 'early pregnancy failure' clinically and sonographically with the initial diagnosis of molar disease being made by the pathologist reporting routine histopathological assessment of products of conception from these failed pregnancies [5].

Whilst distinction between CHM and PHM moles has implications for follow-up counselling and future pregnancies, the most important question to be addressed by the pathologist is simply the recognition of whether there is any kind of suspected hydatidiform mole. This would allow the patient to be registered appropriately and, if required, pathology can be reviewed at a tertiary centre for more specific diagnosis. The majority of hydatidiform mole of either type has no significant clinical sequelae following evacuation. However, around 15% of CHMs and around 1 in 200 PHMs will develop pGTD. In these cases, treatment is usually successful with single-agent chemotherapy, which in the United Kingdom is usually methotrexate. In unresponsive cases, second-line chemotherapy is available and essentially curative [2,3].

GTTs are usually diagnosed in the setting of persistent clinical features according to the size of the tumour and its situation, with abnormal biochemical findings and imaging investigations. The most important issue for the pathologist in this setting is to distinguish between tumours that are choriocarcinomatous, which usually respond well to chemotherapy, and tumours which show an intermediate interstitial trophoblast phenotype, such as PSTT/ETT, which requires surgery as first-line treatment. In some rare cases, it may be difficult to distinguish morphologically between a primary GTT and nongestational malignancies showing trophoblastic differentiation. However, this distinction is important since the prognosis for GTT is significantly better and in such cases definitive diagnosis may require ancillary investigations, in particular, molecular genotyping [6].

PATHOLOGY OF HYDATIDIFORM MOLES

Because of the changes in clinical management noted above, the majority of hydatidiform moles of either type are evacuated in the first trimester of pregnancy, usually around 9–10 weeks of gestation. For this reason, the histopathological findings are different from those described classically in the literature as these are based on cases which were evacuated in the late second trimester. Nevertheless, all hydatidiform moles represent genetically abnormal pregnancies which are characterised by relative overabundance and/or expression of the paternal genome, which leads to abnormal placental development, abnormal or absent fetal development and characteristic abnormal trophoblastic proliferation.

The traditional terminology of CHM versus PHM was primarily based on their microscopic and low-power histological features when traditionally presenting in midgestation, according to whether or not the entire placenta was apparently involved by disease. It is now recognised that PHMs and CHMs are genetically distinct entities with characteristic and distinct histopathological features.

Complete hydatidiform moles

These are abnormal diploid conceptions with the normal number of chromosomes but in which the entire chromosome complement derives from the sperm, to which there is no maternal contribution. In the vast majority of cases, this occurs from a single sperm following endospermic reduplication after fertilisation of an anucleate oocyte [7]. CHMs are characterised by diffuse abnormal villous morphological features with associated abnormal trophoblast proliferation and absence of significant fetal development [8,9]. Villi demonstrate characteristic 'budding' architecture, with myxoid or mucoid stromal appearances and prominent stromal karyorrhexis. At early gestations, blood vessels are often present within the villi, although nucleated red cells are extremely rare, since villous vasculogenesis initially occurs independently of fetal circulation. Trophoblast hyperplasia is characteristically circumferential (i.e. no longer confined to one pole of the villus), with multilayering and pleomorphism (**Figure 7.1**). Note that in early pregnancy, abnormal trophoblast proliferation even in CHM does not affect all of the villi. However, the stromal features such as karyorrhexis are usually marked in all villi, whereas abnormal trophoblast hyperplasia affects only around 30% of villi at this stage of pregnancy [10].

In the majority of cases, the morphological features of early CHMs are distinctive, and the diagnosis can often be made either at low power magnification or on the basis of just one or two villi. Rarely, there are cases with unusual features at very early gestations, and in these immunohistochemical staining with p57KIP2 is extremely useful since this marker is present in the nucleus of all cells which express the maternal genome [11]. In usual practice, CHM is excluded by the presence of villous trophoblast positive nuclear p57KIP2 immunoreactivity in the majority of cells, and confirmed by the absence of such reactivity. Nevertheless, there are rare situations, such as CHM mosaicism and specific chromosomal deletions, where this is not the case; however, such cases are exceptionally rare, see below. Note that even with CHM, there is normal nuclear expression of p57KIP2 in extravillous trophoblast fragments, a finding which is helpful as a normal internal control [12].

Partial hydatidiform mole

These are abnormal triploid conceptions in which the additional chromosomal component also derives from the sperm, usually due to dispermic fertilisation of an apparently normal oocyte [7]. In this setting, there is relative overexpression of the paternal genome although there is also some maternal genome expression; hence, the histological features differ slightly from CHM, which are purely androgenetic. In PHM, the villi also show dysmorphic

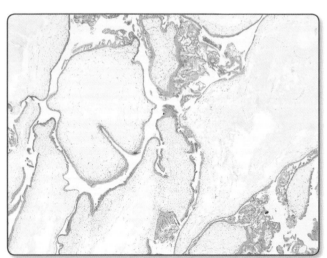

Figure 7.1 Photomicrograph of a first trimester genetically confirmed complete hydatidiform mole demonstrating villous hydropic change and increased stromal cellularity. Abnormally distributed trophoblast hyperplasia is present; note that in early gestations the extent of trophoblast proliferation may be highly variable even in complete moles (H&E, original magnification ×40).

features, such as irregular outlines and trophoblastic pseudoinclusions, and focal abnormal trophoblast hyperplasia [8,9]. In early pregnancy, there are no two clear populations of villi, rather there are villi present ranging from morphologically normal to markedly hydropic and abnormal. Individual villi show characteristic indented, irregular profiles with, often, numerous associated pseudoinclusions. The stroma is relatively unremarkable containing vessels with nucleated red blood cells. Trophoblast hyperplasia is nonpolar and demonstrates mild multilayering, with a typical 'lace-like' or vacuolated appearance and mild pleomorphism (**Figure 7.2**). However, the proportion of villi affected by such changes is reduced compared to CHM and the changes themselves are often more subtle. For example, at around 10 weeks of gestation, pathological trophoblast hyperplasia affects only around 5% of PHM villi [10]. For this reason, the diagnosis of PHM on morphological grounds alone can sometimes be extremely difficult, particularly when the differential diagnosis is a nonmolar. Indeed, chromosomally abnormal pregnancy loss may also show similar villous architectural features but without the characteristic molar type 'lacy' or 'vacuolated' trophoblast proliferation. Furthermore, since changes in PHM may be focal, in cases with limited material and only scanty villi present, it is impossible to exclude PHM with certainty on morphological grounds alone due to these sampling issues.

Immunohistochemical reactivity is not useful in the diagnosis of PHM. P57KIP2 positivity can distinguish CHM from PHM. Although this is usually apparent from the morphological features, it is of no value in distinguishing PHM from nonmolar miscarriage.

Unusual situations – BiCHM, CHM mosaics and twin moles

Although the above criteria hold true for almost all cases likely to be encountered by general histopathologists, it is now increasingly recognised that a minority of cases of hydatidiform moles demonstrate slightly atypical features corresponding to specific subtypes or clinical situations. In all these settings, the most important factor is the recognition of possible CHM, and that further investigation should be performed at a tertiary centre if required.

Biparental familial complete hydatidiform mole (BiCHM) is now recognised as a familial genetic disorder of fertilisation in families with a history of multiple molar

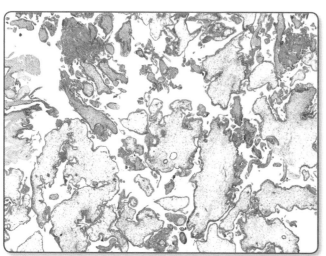

Figure 7.2 Photomicrograph of a first trimester genetically confirmed partial hydatidiform mole demonstrating patchy villous hydropic change, with marked villous dysmorphism (irregularly shaped villi with trophoblastic pseudoinclusions). In partial mole, the extent of trophoblast proliferation may be highly variable and no diagnostic trophoblast hyperplasia is present in this field (H&E, original magnification ×20)

pregnancies, usually recurrent CHM [13]. The underlying abnormality appears to be a maternal defect in control of imprinting such that fertilisation apparently occurs as normal, with the conceptus having one maternal and one paternal copy of the genome, but only the paternal genes are expressed, resulting in molar pregnancy [14]. The histological findings of such cases are often indistinguishable from typical androgenetic CHM, but in some cases the pathological features may be subtly different and less marked, and particularly in the appropriate clinical context, may raise the possibility of this condition [15]. The diagnosis requires the combination of molecular genetic testing, demonstrating an apparently normal biparental genotype, along with reliable histopathological examination including abnormal P57KIP2 immunostaining which supports a diagnosis of CHM. The gene most commonly implicated in such families is *NLRP7*, but a large range of mutations have been described, often unique to individual families [16]. Patients present with many pregnancy losses, most of which are molar, with only rare livebirths reported. Oocyte donation may allow such patients to achieve a normal pregnancy [17].

There are also two scenarios in which products of conception may appear to demonstrate clearly a mixture of villi with morphological features and immunostaining characteristics that are typical of CHM and other areas which appear to be nonmolar. These represent mosaic CHM, and more commonly dizygotic twin pregnancies in which one twin is a CHM and the other is nonmolar. Twin CHMs, usually, clearly demonstrate two geographically separate villous populations, whereas with mosaic CHM the normal and molar villi are more diffusely intermixed [18,19].

NONMOLAR MISCARRIAGE

There may be significant overlap between histopathological features of nonmolar early pregnancy failure and early hydatidiform moles; in particular, hydropic change is a poor discriminatory factor in early gestation where nonmolar miscarriages may exhibit greater villous hydrops than hydatidiform moles. In the majority of cases, an experienced pathologist can differentiate between these groups based on the other villous morphologic features and the presence or absence of abnormal trophoblast hyperplasia, but in some cases this distinction is impossible considering morphology alone.

In general, compared to PHM, nonmolar hydropic miscarriages show more uniform villous size, regardless of the extent of placental hydrops which are generally represented by regular (rounded) villous outlines and fewer trophoblastic inclusions (**Figure 7.3**). Chromosomally abnormal, but nonmolar, products, such as fetal trisomies, however can show almost identical villous structural features to PHM, the distinction being that only PHMs show characteristic abnormal trophoblast hyperplasia. However, abnormal trophoblast 'sprouting' can also be recognised in cases of other chromosomal abnormalities and in some cases it is impossible to exclude PHM without ancillary investigations [8,9]. In such cases, molecular genotyping reliably provides the diagnosis (as it does with almost all cases of hydatidiform moles). However, routine use of molecular testing is not cost effective, since hCG surveillance to ensure that levels return to normal will detect all cases of pGTD; most nonmolar cases are associated with a rapid fall in serum hCG concentration and prolonged follow-up is therefore not required [20,21].

Finally, another specific condition known as placental mesenchymal dysplasia (PMD) may be confused with PHM, although in this case, it usually occurs in later pregnancy.

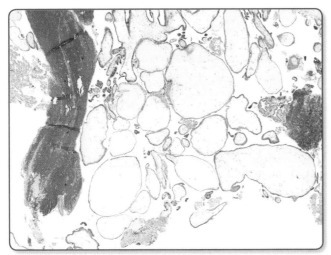

Figure 7.3 Photomicrograph of a first trimester nonmolar hydropic miscarriage demonstrating marked villous hydropic change, but with generally regular and round villous outlines, reduced stromal cellularity and no abnormal trophoblast proliferation (H&E, original magnification ×40)

In PMD, an infant is delivered in association with a macroscopically or sonographically abnormal placenta, which demonstrates prominent chorionic plate vessels and scattered parenchymal cysts throughout the placenta. Histologically, the hydropic villi are characteristically stem villi, and there is no trophoblast hyperplasia. It has been proposed that PMD represents a biparental/androgenetic mosaic condition, the stromal cells being androgenetic, but with no increased risk of pGTD development [21,22].

PATHOLOGY OF GTTs

Overview

The diagnosis of GTT is usually made in two settings: first, small biopsies or curettage specimens in patients with vaginal bleeding and/or a uterine mass, and secondly in resection specimens, usually hysterectomies, for suspected tumour. Obviously, as with other tumour types, a specific diagnosis is usually much easier to make when the entire hysterectomy specimen is available for examination. GTTs are usually described as if the various subtypes are entirely distinct but a single tumour may show areas with overlapping features including any combination of the specific types noted below. Furthermore, the morphological phenotype of a resected tumour may be significantly modified by the effects of preceding chemotherapy. For example, post-treatment CC may show dominant mononuclear cytotrophoblast-like features.

If a resection specimen is received from a suspected GTT, it is extremely important that the specimen is thoroughly sampled, particularly if no lesion was identified on presurgical imaging but a suspected diagnosis has been made on a curettage specimen. In such cases, the lesion may be small and difficult to identify by naked eyes, and even with obvious tumours, the microscopic extent of disease may be significantly greater than that estimated macroscopically. This is especially the case with PSTT/ETT. In the majority of cases following resection, the diagnosis is straightforward but in cases in which the morphological or immunohistochemical features are unusual, or in a patient of unusual age or other demographic features, the possibility of a nongestational malignancy showing trophoblastic differentiation should always be considered. In these cases, molecular genetic testing is indicated to resolve any uncertainty.

All GTTs are forms of carcinoma derived from trophoblast and hence express cytokeratins, variable hCG and inhibins. Further immunostaining is useful to determine the type of extravillous differentiation in PSTT/ETT.

CHORIOCARCINOMA

This is a malignant GTT in which the predominant phenotype is that of villous-type trophoblast, almost always showing at least focally a biphasic- or triphasic-type pattern with areas recapitulating the phenotypes of cytotrophoblast and syncytiotrophoblast, with or without intermediate trophoblast (**Figure 7.4**) [1]. In most cases, there is invasion, necrosis and haemorrhage, and the trophoblast shows marked pleomorphism. In cases which have already undergone chemotherapy prior to resection, the pleomorphic component may show significant reduction and the tumour may show a relatively monomorphic phenotype. Since the trophoblast is of villous type, the serum hCG concentrations are markedly increased in cases of CC.

In resection or metastatic specimens, the diagnosis of CC is usually uncomplicated but the diagnosis should be made with caution in curettage specimens. Evacuations may show fragments of pleomorphic trophoblast only, in the absence of villi or other clinical or biochemical features. Since florid atypical trophoblast may be associated with CHM even in the absence of CC and, unless there is clear invasion, the diagnosis of malignancy in this context should only be made with other clinical, biochemical and imaging characteristics.

Immunostaining of CC reveals diffuse expression of AE1/3 and inhibin, ki67 index >90% and patchy diffuse hCG expression [1].

PLACENTAL SITE TROPHOBLASTIC TUMOUR AND EPITHELIOID TROPHOBLASTIC TUMOUR

These represent malignant GTT tumours with predominant differentiation towards intermediate interstitial trophoblast recapitulating the implanting conceptus (some

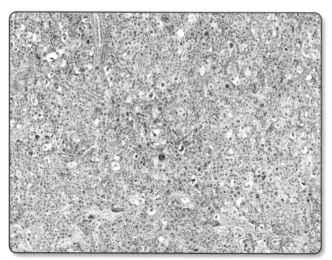

Figure 7.4 Photomicrograph of gestational choriocarcinoma demonstrating sheets of highly pleomorphic malignant cells, with features recapitulating cytotrophoblast and syncytiotrophoblast-like areas. (H&E, original magnification ×40)

authors distinguish between placental and chorionic types). Therefore, they usually manifest as uterine poorly circumscribed tumours with extensive single-cell infiltration peripherally. The tumour is composed of sheets, cords, nests and single cells of relatively monomorphic trophoblast with clear eosinophilic cytoplasm, with pleomorphism, but mild compared to CC (**Figure 7.5**). The features are variable, but there are often extensive areas of associated hyalinisation and/or necrosis, with viable tumour peripherally [1].

The distinction between PSTT and ETT can often be based on the overall architecture and degree of hyalinisation [more extensive in ETT with central eosinophilic material (**Figure 7.6**)], along with their immunohistochemical profile (see below). However, from a practical perspective, the clinical significance of this distinction is probably minimal and both PSTT and ETT are likely to represent different phenotypes of a similar tumour. It should also be noted that it is now recognised that some cases of PSTT and ETT have peripheral areas resembling either typical placental site nodule (PSN) or atypical PSN (with increased cellularity, mild pleomorphism and raised ki67 index), suggesting that

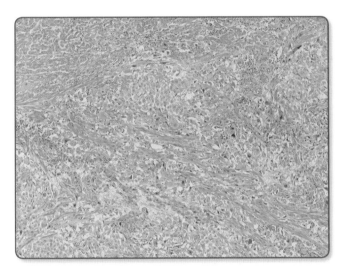

Figure 7.5 Photomicrograph of placental site trophoblastic tumour demonstrating myometrial invasion by sheets of monomorphic cells with eosinophilic cytoplasm morphologically recapitulating implantation site extravillous interstitial trophoblast. (H&E, original magnification ×40)

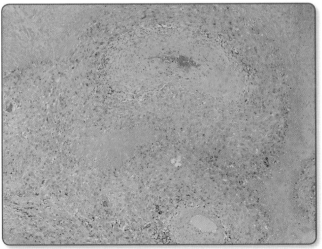

Figure 7.6 Photomicrograph of epithelioid trophoblastic tumour, a variant of placental site trophoblastic tumour, demonstrating areas of hyalinisation and relatively bland, ovoid tumour cells, recapitulating extravillous interstitial trophoblast. (H&E, original magnification ×40)

PSTT/ETT may be derived from such precursor lesions. In a curettage specimen, the presence of a PSN should be specifically highlighted, since in around 15% of cases such findings are associated with coexisting or subsequent development of PSTT/ETT [23].

Immunostaining of PSTT and ETT reveals diffuse expression of cytokeratin, inhibin and HLAG, with only focal hCG expression. PSTT characteristically expresses diffuse human placental lactogen (hPL) and CD146 (Mel-CAM), whereas ETT diffusely expresses p63 and cyclin E [24,25].

FUTURE DEVELOPMENTS

Currently, CHM and PHM all require hCG surveillance in order to allow early detection of pGTD and hence cure with minimal chemotherapy. Whilst the rates of pGTD are markedly increased following hydatidiform moles compared to a nonmolar pregnancy, the majority of hydatidiform moles, even CHM, will resolve spontaneously following evacuation. Diagnosis of hydatidiform moles is now reliable and hence current research efforts focus on determining prognosis and the need for subsequent chemotherapy at the time of hydatidiform moles detection, rather than simply instituting hCG surveillance for all cases. Unfortunately, at present, despite many studies attempting to relate morphological and immunohistochemical findings to outcome, there are no reliable markers capable of predicting subsequent behaviour [26]. Since the risk of pGTD is not related to gestational age at evacuation of hydatidiform moles [27], it is likely that determination of pGTD risk is based on genetic factors established early in their development, and future detailed molecular genotyping may allow individualised risk stratification and hence personalised medicine and treatment of GTD [28].

ACKNOWLEDGEMENTS

NJS is an NIHR Senior Investigator and part supported by the NIHR GOSH Biomedical Research Centre and GOSHCC. NJS has no conflict of interest and no commercial or financial interests.

Key points for clinical practice

- The majority of hydatidiform moles will present as vaginal bleeding in early pregnancy or early pregnancy failure.
- Cases of hydatidiform mole, especially partial mole, may show no molar features sonographically or clinically and hence the first suspicion of the diagnosis may be made following routine histological evaluation of products of conception.
- The risk of pGTD is increased following the diagnosis of partial or complete hydatidiform mole, and all cases should undergo hCG surveillance.
- Distinction of partial mole from non-molar miscarriage may be impossible on morphology alone and ancillary investigations such as ploidy or molecular studies may be required.
- Any hCG producing tumour in a women of childbearing age should be considered GTT until proven otherwise.
- Tumours may sometimes demonstrate overlapping features between the phenotypes of CC, PSTT and ETT.

REFERENCES

1. Hui P, Baergen R, Cheung ANY, et al. Gestational trophoblastic diseases. In: Kurman RJ, Carcangiu ML, Herrington CS, Young RH (eds.), WHO classification of tumours of female reproductive organs. Lyon: IARC, 2014:155–167.
2. Seckl MJ, Sebire NJ, Berkowitz RS. Gestational trophoblastic disease. Lancet 2010; 376:717–729.
3. Sebire NJ, Seckl MJ. Gestational trophoblastic disease: current management of hydatidiform mole. BMJ 2008; 337:a1193.
4. Schmid P, Nagai Y, Agarwal R, et al. Prognostic markers and long-term outcome of placental-site trophoblastic tumours: a retrospective observational study. Lancet 2009; 374:48–55.
5. Fowler DJ, Lindsay I, Seckl MJ, et al. Routine pre-evacuation ultrasound diagnosis of hydatidiform mole: experience of more than 1000 cases from a regional referral center. Ultrasound Obstet Gynecol 2006; 27:56–60.
6. Fisher RA, Savage PM, MacDermott C, et al. The impact of molecular genetic diagnosis on the management of women with hCG-producing malignancies. Gynecol Oncol 2007; 107:413–419.
7. Bestor TH, Bourc'his D. Genetics and epigenetics of hydatidiform moles. Nat Genet 2006; 38:274–276.
8. Sebire NJ, Makrydimas G, Agnantis NJ, et al. Updated diagnostic criteria for partial and complete hydatidiform moles in early pregnancy. Anticancer Res 2003; 23:1723–1728.
9. Sebire NJ. Histopathological diagnosis of hydatidiform mole: contemporary features and clinical implications. Fetal Pediatr Pathol 2010; 29:1–16.
10. Petts G, Fisher RA, Short D, et al. Histopathological and immunohistochemical features of early hydatidiform mole in relation to subsequent development of persistent gestational trophoblastic disease. J Reprod Med 2014; 59:213–220.
11. Fukunaga M. Immunohistochemical characterization of p57(KIP2) expression in early hydatidiform moles. Hum Pathol 2002; 33:1188–1192.
12. McConnell TG, Murphy KM, Hafez M, et al. Diagnosis and subclassification of hydatidiform moles using p57 immunohistochemistry and molecular genotyping: validation and prospective analysis in routine and consultation practice settings with development of an algorithmic approach. Am J Surg Pathol 2009; 33:805–817.
13. Fisher RA, Hodges MD, Newlands ES. Familial recurrent hydatidiform mole: a review. J Reprod Med 2004; 49:595–601.
14. Hayward BE, De Vos M, Talati N, et al. Genetic and epigenetic analysis of recurrent hydatidiform mole. Hum Mutat 2009; 30:629–639.
15. Sebire NJ, Savage PM, Seckl MJ, et al. Histopathological features of biparental complete hydatidiform moles in women with NLRP7 mutations. Placenta 2013; 34:50–56.
16. Wang CM, Dixon PH, Decordova S, et al. Identification of 13 novel NLRP7 mutations in 20 families with recurrent hydatidiform mole; missense mutations cluster in the leucine-rich region. J Med Genet 2009; 46:569–575.
17. Fisher RA, Lavery SA, Carby A, et al. What a difference an egg makes. Lancet 2011; 378:1974.
18. Makrydimas G, Sebire NJ, Thornton SE, et al. Complete hydatidiform mole and normal live birth: a novel case of confined placental mosaicism: case report. Hum Reprod 2002; 17:2459–2463.
19. Sebire NJ, Foskett M, Paradinas FJ, et al. Outcome of twin pregnancies with complete hydatidiform mole and healthy co-twin. Lancet 2002; 359:2165–2166.
20. Banet N, DeScipio C, Murphy KM, et al. Characteristics of hydatidiform moles: analysis of a prospective series with p57 immunohistochemistry and molecular genotyping. Mod Pathol 2014; 27:238–254.
21. Fisher RA, Tommasi A, Short D, et al. Clinical utility of selective molecular genotyping for diagnosis of partial hydatidiform mole: a retrospective study from a regional trophoblastic disease unit. J Clin Pathol 2014; 67:980–984.
22. Kaiser-Rogers KA, McFadden DE, Livasy CA, et al. Androgenetic/biparental mosaicism causes placental mesenchymal dysplasia. J Med Genet 2006; 43:187–192.
23. Kaur B, Short D, Fisher RA, et al. Atypical placental site nodule (APSN) and association with malignant gestational trophoblastic disease: a clinicopathologic study of 21 cases. Int J Gynecol Pathol 2015; 34:152–158.
24. Shih IM, Kurman RJ. The pathology of intermediate trophoblastic tumors and tumor-like lesions. Int J Gynecol Pathol 2001; 20:31–47.
25. Shih IM, Kurman RJ. p63 expression is useful in the distinction of epithelioid trophoblastic and placental site trophoblastic tumors by profiling trophoblastic subpopulations. Am J Surg Pathol 2004; 28:1177–1183.

26. Sebire NJ, Seckl MJ. Immunohistochemical staining for diagnosis and prognostic assessment of hydatidiform moles: current evidence and future directions. J Reprod Med 2010; 55:236–246.

27. Seckl MJ, Dhillon T, Dancey G, et al. Increased gestational age at evacuation of a complete hydatidiform mole: does it correlate with increased risk of requiring chemotherapy? J Reprod Med 2004; 49:527–530.

28. Blay JY, Lacombe D, Meunier F, et al. Personalised medicine in oncology: questions for the next 20 years. Lancet Oncol 2012; 13:448–449.

Chapter 8

Embryonal brain tumours in children

Thomas S Jacques, Antony J Michalski

INTRODUCTION

Epidemiology

Cancer in childhood is rare with only 1:600 children developing a malignancy by 15 years of age. From 20 to 25% of childhood malignancies are primary tumours of the central nervous system (CNS). This equates to 2.4 cases per 100,000 children per year with a male to female ratio of 1.1:1. Unlike adults, the majority of CNS malignancies in childhood are primary brain tumours. While CNS metastases may occur from rhabdoid tumours, sarcomas and neuroblastomas, they are rare. Of primary CNS tumours in childhood, low-grade astrocytomas are the most common but of the high-grade tumours the largest group are the embryonal tumours.

Outcome

With improvements in therapy for leukaemia, CNS tumours are now the most common cause of death for children with malignancy. Planning therapy is complicated by the on-going maturation of the CNS. 40% of CNS tumours in childhood arise in children under 5 years of age and these young children are particularly vulnerable to the deleterious effects of the tumour, hydrocephalus, surgery, chemotherapy and particularly radiotherapy [1]. Radiotherapy is a key component of therapy for embryonal tumours but, when administered to the neuraxis in children, causes profound defects in intellectual function and performance status. The younger the children, the more severe the late effects. The challenge is to differentiate those children who have good risk disease in whom therapy can be reduced, thereby sparing them some of the late effects of therapy, from those with a poor outcome in whom therapy needs to be changed or intensified.

The challenges of stratified medicine for children

Most children with CNS tumours are treated on national or international clinical trials. These studies define the eligible population on the basis of age, stage and histology

Thomas S Jacques MA MB BChir PhD MRCP FRCPath UCL Institute of Child Health and Great Ormond Street Hospital for Children NHS Foundation Trust, London, UK

Antony J Michalski MB ChB PhD FRCPCH UCL Institute of Child Health and Great Ormond Street Hospital for Children NHS Foundation Trust London, UK

and there is central review of pathology and radiology to ensure that the groups are homogeneous. Retrospective analysis has led to the identification of subgroups with differing outcomes. This process has led to the definition of risk stratification based on age, stage, histology and molecular features. The difficulty is that splitting already rare diseases into multiple subgroups creates challenges in clinical trial design. Classical trial design with randomisation of large numbers of patients will be impossible within a realistic time frame even with international collaboration. Novel statistical designs (e.g. Bayesian methodologies) are being introduced to try and run studies that produce credible results within acceptable time periods.

MEDULLOBLASTOMA

Medulloblastoma are embryonal tumours of the cerebellum and are the commonest embryonal tumour of the brain.

Clinical features

Childhood CNS tumours present late, with an average delay of 9 weeks from first symptom to diagnosis. The symptoms mimic those of more common, benign conditions and are easily misinterpreted. A recent meta-analysis of presenting signs and symptoms has led to guidance on reducing the interval to diagnosis [2]. Cerebellar tumours present with ataxia often manifested as decreased school performance or 'clumsiness,' and ocular signs, e.g. nystagmus or squint. The development of hydrocephalus leads to early morning vomiting, headache, irritability and drowsiness. 35% of children with medulloblastoma have metastatic disease at diagnosis, usually identified on MRI as part of the initial diagnostic staging or on cerebrospinal fluid (CSF) cytology. Metastatic stage is determined by the modified Chang criteria with M0 being no metastases, M1 disease identified on CSF cytology alone, M2 being metastatic disease in the brain, M3 is disease in the spine and M4 is distant disease outside the CNS.

Histology

This tumour is composed of sheets of hyperchromatic primitive cells with angular or rounded nuclei and minimal cytoplasm. The tumour may have a diffuse or nodular architecture. The cells show varying degrees of cytological anaplasia. There may be infiltration of the adjacent leptomeninges, associated with desmoplasia. Homer Wright (neuroblastic) rosettes consist of a small circular arrangement of tumour cells around neuropil without a lumen. However, they may be absent and cannot be relied on for diagnosis.

Immunohistochemistry shows evidence of neuronal differentiation (often best shown by synaptophysin) and in most cases, a lack of glial differentiation. Immunohistochemistry should be considered to exclude atypical teratoid/rhabdoid tumour and embryonal tumour with multilayered rosettes (ETMR) (discussed below).

Subtypes of medulloblastoma

Medulloblastoma can be classified both by histology and by molecular profiling. Clinically, the most important histological forms to differentiate are the classic, nodular/desmoplastic and large cell/anaplastic, because these have different clinical outcomes and may be offered different adjuvant therapy.

In addition, there are four molecular types [3]; SHH, WNT, Groups 3 and 4. These represent four broad groups within which it is anticipated that there are sub-groups. The first two are named after the major signalling pathways implicated in those tumours (sonic hedgehog (SHH) and WNT/β-catenin (WNT)). Not only do these tumours differ according to the signalling pathways but they probably arise from different precursor cells in different parts of the brain [4]. This suggests that they are biologically distinct types of tumours. Not surprisingly therefore, they have different clinical features and outcomes.

These are some correlations between the histological subtype and the molecular subtype. For example, nodular/desmoplastic medulloblastomas are molecularly of the SHH subtype. The correlation is not absolute (e.g. not all SHH medulloblastomas are nodular/desmoplastic). Furthermore, there are additional molecular changes that are prognostic (e.g. *MYC* or *MYCN* amplification) that can occur in multiple molecular subtypes. Therefore, a diagnosis of medulloblastoma needs a layered report consisting of the histological subtype, the molecular subtype, and any additional molecular findings. It should be noted that the interaction of clinical, molecular and histological risk factors is incompletely understood.

Methods for molecular subtyping

Determining the molecular subtype is important because the different tumours have different clinical outcomes (e.g. the WNT subgroup tumours have an excellent prognosis) and because targeted treatments are becoming available (e.g. the use of SHH pathway inhibitors). However, the optimal method of determining the subtype in routine clinical practice is uncertain. A variety of techniques have been proposed including methylation arrays, immunohistochemistry and gene expression panels [5]. In some cases, a single test is regarded as diagnostic (e.g. the demonstration of a pathogenic mutation in the β-catenin gene (*CTNNB1*) is regarded as diagnostic of the WNT subgroup) whereas for other subtypes (e.g. SHH), in particular where specific treatments are proposed, two tests may be advisable.

Histological types of medulloblastoma

Classic medulloblastoma

Classic medulloblastoma are characterised by diffuse sheets of primitive cells without significant nodule formation and without significant anaplasia or large cell change. There may be desmoplasia but this is not associated with significant nodule formation. Similarly, there may be focal or mild anaplasia but this is not the predominant feature. However, the degree of anaplasia that is permissible in this form is not well defined.

Anaplastic/large cell

Anaplastic medulloblastoma is characterised by extensive and prominent cytological anaplasia and is associated with a poorer survival than classic medulloblastoma. The cells show increased mitoses, apoptosis, size, pleomorphism, and often, nuclear wrapping (**Figure 8.1**). The latter is wrapping of one nucleus, almost entirely, around the nucleus of another cell.

Large cell medulloblastoma is characterised by cells with larger vesicular nuclei with distinct nucleoli (**Figure 8.2**). These tumours usually show significant anaplasia and there is significant overlap between anaplastic and large cell subtypes of medulloblastoma. As they

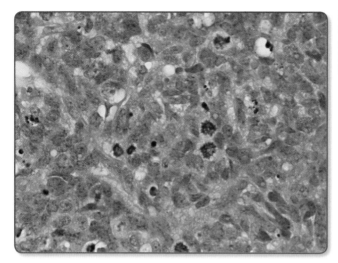

Figure 8.1 Anaplastic medulloblastoma characterised by pleomorphic, moulded nuclei with frequent mitoses and apoptotic bodies.

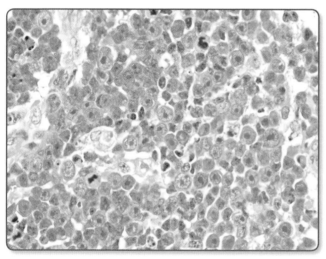

Figure 8.2 Large cell medulloblastoma characterised by large vesicular nuclei and large nucleoli. There is often severe anaplasia.

have a similar poor prognosis, a distinction is often not made and the tumour designated large cell/anaplastic (LCA) medulloblastoma.

It is broadly agreed that very focal anaplasia or relatively mild anaplasia is insufficient but the decision of when the anaplasia is sufficient to warrant a diagnosis of the anaplastic subtype is subjective and poorly defined. Repeated studies have shown the prognostic significance of this subtype but few have addressed how to define the limits of anaplasia in routine clinical practice. In most centres, children with anaplastic medulloblastoma will be offered significantly escalated adjuvant therapy. Therefore, care is required if the only poor prognostic feature is anaplasia.

Desmoplastic/nodular

Desmoplastic/nodular medulloblastoma (DN) is defined by the presence of nodules ('pale islands') of better-differentiated tumour cells and neuropil, surrounded by closely packed cells with poorer differentiation. Within the nodules, there is no significant reticulin deposition but the internodular regions show extensive reticulin deposition (**Figure 8.3**). These tumours are typically of the SHH-subtype. They are generally associated with a better prognosis than classic medulloblastoma. This is particularly the case in children <3 years of age [6].

Medulloblastoma with extensive nodularity

These tumours demonstrate extensive nodularity in which much of the tumour consists of the intra-nodular areas with sparse internodular areas (**Figure 8.4**). The shape of nodules are much more pleomorphic than in more conventional DN medulloblastoma. The cells within the nodules are relatively well differentiated with a neurocytic morphology and expression of mature neuronal markers. The tumour cells may stream, forming lines within the nodules. Medulloblastoma with extensive nodularity typically occur in young children

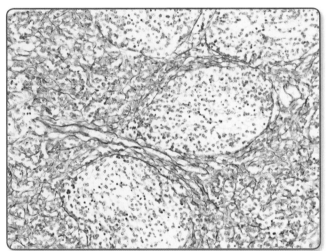

Figure 8.3 Nodular/desmoplastic medulloblastoma showing a typical nodular pattern with desmoplasia in the internodular regions (reticulin stain).

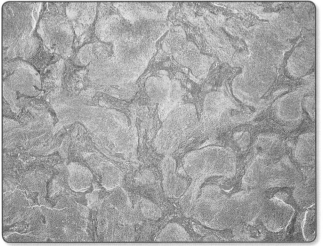

Figure 8.4 Medulloblastoma with extensive nodularity consist mostly of nodules, many of which have unusual and pleomorphic shapes.

and infants and often show typically radiological appearances ('bunch of grapes') on MRI. They are associated with an excellent prognosis with current treatment and there is considerable interest in reducing adjuvant treatment for these children.

Biphasic medulloblastoma

These tumours show similar histological features to the desmoplastic/nodular form of medulloblastoma, in that they have 'pale' nodules. However, in contrast to desmoplastic/nodular medulloblastoma, biphasic tumours lack significant desmoplasia (as demonstrated by reticulin staining) in the internodular areas. Ellison and colleagues showed that the clinical and molecular features of these cases more closely resemble classic or anaplastic medulloblastoma than desmoplastic/nodular medulloblastoma [6].

Medulloblastoma with melanotic or myogenic differentiation

Medulloblastomas may show divergent differentiation. Two forms of differentiation are well recognised: melanotic and myogenic differentiation. However, more diverse differentiation (e.g. chondroid) may be seen. These are relatively rare tumours, and therefore the clinical significance of divergent differentiation is uncertain.

Molecular types of medulloblastoma

WNT-medulloblastoma

WNT-subgroup medulloblastoma are characterised by activation of the WNT-signalling pathway usually due to activating mutations in the β-catenin gene, leading to nuclear localisation of the β-catenin. This subgroup is associated with an excellent prognosis in children [7]. With current treatment protocols, over 95% of patients are alive at 5 years. The significance of WNT subgroup medulloblastoma in adults is less certain and there is evidence that they do not show the same prognostic advantage as seen in children.

The most frequent genetic alteration in WNT subgroup medulloblastoma is a point mutation in exon 3 of the *CTNNB1* gene that encodes for β-catenin. The mutations prevent the phosphorylation of β-catenin that normally leads to its degradation. Therefore, β-catenin becomes stabilised and accumulates in the cytoplasm and nucleus. The nuclear accumulation leads to increased transcription of β-catenin targets. Demonstration of a *CTNNB1* mutation in a medulloblastoma is regarded as sufficient for diagnosis of a WNT subgroup medulloblastoma. Monosomy for chromosome 6 is a frequent finding in WNT subgroup medulloblastoma and may also be used to provide molecular evidence of WNT subgrouping.

β-catenin immunohistochemistry shows nuclear reactivity in WNT subgroup medulloblastoma. Furthermore, the presence of β-catenin nuclear reactivity is predictive of a good prognosis. Assessment of nuclear β-catenin is not always straightforward as assessing nuclear localisation may be difficult and the extent of nuclear localisation may vary considerably (>10% positive nuclei is strongly associated with WNT subgroup medulloblastomas but <10% is more variable). Therefore, if reduced treatment is being contemplated, confirmation by a molecular technique (e.g. *CTNNB1* sequencing or monosomy 6) is recommended.

SHH-medulloblastoma

SHH-medulloblastomas are defined by activation of the sonic hedgehog signalling pathway. SHH subtype medulloblastoma show a diverse range of clinical outcomes.

Some patients, particularly infants with DN medulloblastomas are associated with a good prognosis, whereas those patients with SHH medulloblastomas harbouring *TP53* mutations have a poor prognosis.

TP53 mutations

TP53 mutations are present in 10–20% of WNT and SHH medulloblastoma and very rarely in the other subtypes [8]. In WNT subgroup tumours, the presence of *TP53* mutations has no significant effect on survival. In contrast, in SHH medulloblastoma, patients with mutated *TP53* have a significantly poorer outcome than those with wild type *TP53*. This suggests that testing for *TP53* mutations in SHH group medulloblastoma should identify patients with high-risk disease.

Furthermore, about half of patients with SHH medulloblastoma and tumour *TP53* mutations were found in one study, to have germ-line mutations [8]. This suggests that this group may require altered treatment due to the risks of secondary tumours following radiotherapy. Furthermore, they require genetic counselling because of the possibility of the family harbouring a cancer predisposition.

MYC/MYCN amplification

Many studies have shown that amplification of *MYC* group genes (*MYC* and *MYCN*) is associated with a worse prognosis and examination of these genes is a standard part of risk stratification [9].

CSF cytology

Cytological examination of CSF is a routine part of the staging of medulloblastoma. Samples are taken 2–3 weeks after surgery due to the concern that surgery releases cells into the CSF that may not have metastatic potential. CSF cytology is of low sensitivity compared to MRI for detecting dissemination but there is a poor correlation between MRI and CSF cytology. Therefore, CSF cytology may identify a group of metastatic tumours that wouldn't be recognised by MRI alone [10,11].

Relapsed medulloblastoma

Patients with relapsed medulloblastoma have a poor prognosis but the rate of decline is very variable and there are few data to indicate what will predict the outcome after relapse. It will be very important to understand the biology of this untreatable disease. There is evidence that molecular but not necessarily histological subtype is maintained at relapse. Furthermore, there are data that indicate that at relapse, a subpopulation of tumours emerge that have combined *TP53* and *MYC* abnormalities [12]. Importantly this group of patients has a very short survival compared to other relapsed patients. This suggests that there may be a role for re-biopsy and molecular pathology in determining the outcome for patients at relapse.

ATYPICAL TERATOID/RHABDOID TUMOURS

Atypical teratoid/rhabdoid tumours (ATRT) are the malignant rhabdoid tumours of the CNS. They are defined in the vast majority of cases by biallelic mutations in the *SMARCB1* gene (that encodes for INI1) [13]. There are rare reported cases associated with mutations in the related gene, *SMARCA4* (encoding for BRG1) [14].

Clinical features

ATRTs comprise 1–2% of all CNS tumours in childhood but may form up to 20% of tumours seen in children <3 years of age. Rorke et al [15] published an early series that showed a male to female ratio of 1.9:1 and a median age of diagnosis of 17 months. In younger children, the tumours are more likely to be infratentorial and up to 20% of patients have signs of metastatic disease at diagnosis. Metastatic disease and young age (perhaps due to the avoidance of radiotherapy) are poor prognostic factors. Older children with no metastatic disease, treated with dose intensive alkylator based chemotherapy and radiation therapy can do well (2 year overall survival of 89 ± 11%) but younger children treated without radiation fare very poorly with survival rates of <20% [16].

Rhabdoid predisposition syndrome

In young children, around 35% of patients will carry a constitutional mutation of the *SMARCB1* gene [17]. These children can present with multifocal synchronous or metachronous tumours and their disease carries a particularly poor prognosis with the majority relapsing or progressing on therapy.

Histology

The histology of ATRT is very variable and while they may show typical rhabdoid cells and divergent differentiation, in many cases, this histology demonstrates a primitive malignant tumour without distinctive histological features (**Figure 8.5**). Therefore, the diagnosis should be considered and actively excluded in any malignant CNS tumour in a young child.

Immunophenotype

The key diagnostic feature is the loss of nuclear immunoreactivtiy for INI1 (encoded by *SMARCB1*). The stain is retained in the endothelium and host inflammatory cells, which

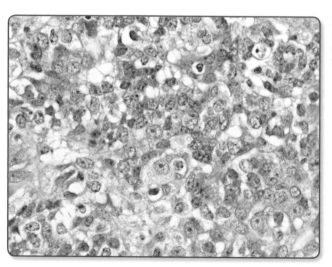

Figure 8.5 Atypical teratoid/ rhabdoid tumour showing variable cytology with some cells with large vesicular nuclei and large nucleoli.

serve as internal controls. Uniform loss of nuclear INI1 amongst tumour cells in a primitive malignant brain tumour is sufficient for diagnosis of an ATRT and is strongly correlated with genetic defects in the *SMARCB1* gene [13]. In the rare cases of *SMARCA4* mutations, BRG1 staining has been reported to be lost [14].

Molecular investigation

A range of defects in the *SMARCB1* gene can be demonstrated in ATRT but are not usually required for the diagnosis. Genetic investigation may be required when the rhabdoid predisposition syndrome is under consideration.

There are data that suggest that ATRT can be subdivided into distinct subtypes based on the molecular profiling and that some of these may relate to clinical outcome [18]. These subtypes have not entered into routine clinical practice.

Differential diagnosis

Within the nervous system, INI1 loss is only described in a small proportion of tumour types. Loss is seen in the rare low grade tumour, the cribriform neuroectodermal tumour [19], some dedifferentiated chordomas [20] and may occur in schwannomatosis [21]. However, due to the distinctive histological features, these tumours do not usually present a significant differential diagnosis.

It is not possible to differentiate routinely on pathological grounds between an ATRT, metastatic rhabdoid tumour (from outside the nervous system) or synchronous tumours (in the brain and outside the nervous system) but this rarely presents a significant clinical question.

INI1 may be lost in a number of nonrhabdoid tumours outside the nervous system [13] but these rarely present a genuine differential diagnosis in the context of a CNS tumour in a child.

EMBRYONAL TUMOURS WITH MULTILAYERED ROSETTES

The term ETMR has been proposed to describe a range of tumours that are unified by amplification of a miRNA cluster on chromosome 19 (*C19MC*) and over-expression of the RNA-binding protein, LIN28a [22,23].

Relation to historical terms

The term embryonal tumour with abundant neuropil and true rosettes (ETANTR) was introduced to describe a tumour with distinctive morphological features: Ependymoblastomous rosettes, characterised by multilayered cells surrounding a lumen, patches of dense cellularity and areas of more differentiated tumour with abundant neuropil. As this tumour has been better characterised and in particular, the distinctive genetic changes that characterise this tumour identified, evidence has accumulated that there are a range of genetically similar embryonal tumours that have traditionally been labelled as ETANTR, ependymoblastoma or medulloepithelioma. This has led to the suggestion that this group of tumours are a single biological entity, embryonal tumour with multilayered rosettes (ETMR) [24].

Histology

The morphology of these tumours varies. They are all embryonal tumours with malignant primitive cells. The presence of multilayered rosettes and the presence of varying cellular density with areas of better differentiated tumour with prominent neuropil are clues to the diagnosis (**Figure 8.6**). However on a biopsy, there may be considerable sampling artefact and the absence of these features does not exclude the diagnosis.

Immunophenotype

The most helpful immunohistochemical feature is the presence of strong cytoplasmic immunoreactivity for Lin28a in a proportion of the tumour cells. However, this is not entirely specific and has been described in ATRT and germ cell tumours.

Molecular diagnosis

Confirmation of the diagnosis can be made by demonstration the amplification of the *C19MC* locus by FISH. There is an associated fusion between the *TTYR1* gene and the *C19MC* region and a downstream overexpression of the DNA methylase, DNMT3B [25].

Clinical outcome

The clinical outcome of ETMR is particularly poor with early progression of disease and death. Survival is very poor indeed and these children warrant novel therapeutic approaches rather than therapy on toxic protocols that are destined to fail.

CNS-PNET/SUPRATENTORIAL PNET

The terms supratentorial primitive neuroectodermal tumour (PNET) and central nervous system primitive neuroectodermal tumour (CNS-PNET) have been used to describe nonmedulloblastoma embryonal tumours of the nervous system. However, the status of this diagnosis is being re-evaluated in the light of molecular data. First a proportion of

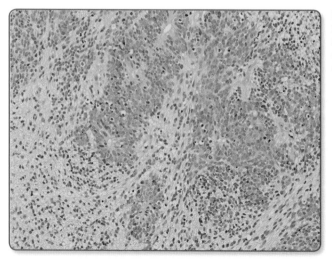

Figure 8.6 Embryonal tumour with multilayered rosettes composed of a mixture of primitive tumour cells, neuropil rich areas and true multilayered rosettes.

CNS-PNETs are now reclassified at ATRT or ETMR. Second, it is likely that a proportion of the remaining tumours are better recognised as high-grade gliomas as defined by their methylation profile and the presence of histone mutations, typically seen in gliomas [26,27]. It is likely that further molecular profiling will redefine the use of this diagnosis.

From a practical point of view when considering this diagnosis, one needs to exclude actively ATRT and ETMR by looking for the expression of INI1 and Lin28a/*C19MC* using immunohistochemistry. Furthermore, the possibility of a high-grade glioma needs to be considered and actively investigated (e.g. immunoreactivity for glial markers and by sequencing the histone genes *H3F3A* and *HIST1H3B* for mutations (K27M and G34) that typify high grade gliomas). This is particularly important as the traditional treatment protocols for CNS-PNET and high-grade glioma are very different and the outcome and treatment-associated morbidity will differ significantly.

PINEOBLASTOMA

Pineoblastomas are high-grade embryonal tumours of the pineal gland. Some patients have germ-line mutations in either the retinoblastoma gene (*RB-1*) or in the *DICER1* gene [28].

Pineoblastoma presents with signs related to the location of the tumour in the upper midbrain, classically with Parinaud's syndrome which is characterised by failure of up-gaze, pupils that react poorly to light but respond to accommodation, nystagmus (retraction or convergence type) and lid retraction. Not all of these signs are present in every case and the syndrome can be seen in patients with other causes of third ventricular dilatation. Hydrocephalus occurs in the majority of patients and may be the presenting complaint. Up to 15% of cases will have signs of metastatic disease within the CNS at diagnosis.

The histology of most pineoblastomas consists of diffuse sheets of hyperchromatic angular nuclei with minimal cytoplasm. Immunohistochemistry shows reactivity for neuronal markers (synaptophysin) but are negative for glial markers. They show retained INI1 staining and lack Lin28a staining.

PITUITARY BLASTOMA

Pituitary blastoma is a rare primitive embryonal tumour of the pituitary gland [29]. It typically presents in the first 2 years of life with Cushing's syndrome, which may be accompanied by ophthalmaplaegia. The histology shows a combination of epithelial structures, small embryonal cells and secretory cells. The latter express synaptophysin and chromogranin and usually at least some express pituitary hormones (typically ACTH). There is a high frequency of germ-line *DICER1* mutations and there may be a history of other tumours that are seen in the *DICER1* predisposition syndrome.

Key points for clinical practice

- Brain tumours are the most common malignancy-related cause of death in children.
- Therapy is complicated by the impact of treatments, particularly radiotherapy, on the developing nervous system.
- Planning treatment represents a balance between maximising survival and causing long-term disability.

- Molecular and pathological stratification is critical in determining the type and intensity of treatment.
- Medulloblastoma, the most common embryonal tumour, can be stratified on the basis of histological and molecular subtypes into high risk disease (anaplastic/large cell, MYC/MYCN amplified) and low risk disease (WNT subtype).
- Classification of other embryonal tumour types by molecular approaches is defining new subtypes with distinct clinical outcomes.

REFERENCES

1. Kiltie AE, Lashford LS. Survival and late effects in medulloblastoma patients treated with craniospinal irradiation under three years old. Med Pediatr Oncol 1997; 28:348–354.
2. Wilne S, Koller K, Collier J, et al. The diagnosis of brain tumours in children: a guideline to assist healthcare professionals in the assessment of children who may have a brain tumour. Arch Dis Child 2010; 95:534–539.
3. Taylor MD, Northcott PA, Korshunov A, et al. Molecular subgroups of medulloblastoma: the current consensus. Acta Neuropathol 2012; 123:465–472.
4. Gibson P, Tong Y, Robinson G, et al. Subtypes of medulloblastoma have distinct developmental origins. Nature 2010; 468:1095–1099.
5. Ellison DW, Dalton J, Kocak M, et al. Medulloblastoma: clinicopathological correlates of SHH, WNT, and non-SHH/WNT molecular subgroups. Acta Neuropathol 2011; 121:381–396.
6. McManamy CS, Pears J, Weston CL, et al. Nodule formation and desmoplasia in medulloblastomas-defining the nodular/desmoplastic variant and its biological behaviour. Brain Pathol 2007; 17:151–164.
7. Stone TJ, Jacques TS. Medulloblastoma: selecting children for reduced treatment. Neuropathology and Applied Neurobiology 2015; 41:106–108.
8. Zhukova N, Ramaswamy V, Remke M, et al. Subgroup-Specific Prognostic Implications of TP53 Mutation in Medulloblastoma. J Clin Oncol 2013; 31:2927–2935.
9. Eberhart CG, Kratz J, Wang Y, et al. Histopathological and molecular prognostic markers in medulloblastoma: c-myc, N-myc, TrkC, and anaplasia. J Neuropathol Exp Neurol 2004; 63:441–449.
10. Cohen NR, Phipps K, Harding B, et al. CSF cytology in paediatric practice: an important staging investigation in the absence of MRI-proven leptomeningeal spread. Neuropathology and Applied Neurobiology 2008; 34:26–46.
11. Meyers SP, Wildenhain SL, Chang JK, et al. Postoperative evaluation for disseminated medulloblastoma involving the spine: contrast-enhanced MR findings, CSF cytologic analysis, timing of disease occurrence, and patient outcomes. AJNR Am J Neuroradiol 2000; 21:1757–1765.
12. Hill RM, Kuijper S, Lindsey JC, et al. Combined MYC and P53 defects emerge at medulloblastoma relapse and define rapidly progressive, therapeutically targetable disease. Cancer Cell 2015; 27:72–84.
13. Margol AS, Judkins AR. Pathology and diagnosis of SMARCB1-deficient tumors. Cancer Genet 2014; 207:358–364.
14. Hasselblatt M, Gesk S, Oyen F, et al. Nonsense mutation and inactivation of SMARCA4 (BRG1) in an atypical teratoid/rhabdoid tumor showing ertained SMARCB1 (INI1) expression. Am J Surg Pathol 2011; 35:933–935.
15. Rorke LB, Packer R, Biegel J. Central nervous system atypical teratoid/rhabdoid tumors of infancy and childhood. J Neurooncol 1995; 24:21–28.
16. Tekautz TM, Fuller CE, Blaney S, et al. Atypical teratoid/rhabdoid tumors (ATRT): improved survival in children 3 years of age and older with radiation therapy and high-dose alkylator-based chemotherapy. J Clin Oncol 2005; 23:1491–1499.
17. Eaton KW, Tooke LS, Wainwright LM, et al. Spectrum of SMARCB1/INI1 mutations in familial and sporadic rhabdoid tumors. Pediatr Blood Cancer 2011; 56:7–15.
18. Torchia J, Picard D, Lafay-Cousin L, et al. Molecular subgroups of atypical teratoid rhabdoid tumours in children: an integrated genomic and clinicopathological analysis. Lancet Oncol 2015; 16:569–582.
19. Hasselblatt M, Oyen F, Gesk S, et al. Cribriform neuroepithelial tumor (CRINET): a nonrhabdoid ventricular tumor with INI1 loss and relatively favorable prognosis. J Neuropathol Exp Neurol 2009; 68:1249–1255.

20. Tirabosco R, Jacques TS, Berisha F, et al. Assessment of integrase interactor 1 (INI-1) expression in primary tumours of bone. Histopathology 2012; 61:1245–1247.
21. Hulsebos TJM, Plomp AS, Wolterman RA, et al. Germline mutation of INI1/SMARCB1 in familial schwannomatosis. Expression of diagnostic neuronal markers and outcome in glioblastoma 2007; 80:805–810.
22. Korshunov A, Ryzhova M, Jones DTW, et al. LIN28A immunoreactivity is a potent diagnostic marker of embryonal tumor with multilayered rosettes (ETMR). Acta Neuropathol 2012; 124:875–881.
23. Korshunov A, Remke M, Gessi M, et al. Focal genomic amplification at 19q13.42 comprises a powerful diagnostic marker for embryonal tumors with ependymoblastic rosettes. Acta Neuropathol 2010; 120:253–260.
24. Spence T, Sin-Chan P, Picard D, et al. CNS-PNETs with C19MC amplification and/or LIN28 expression comprise a distinct histogenetic diagnostic and therapeutic entity. Acta Neuropathol 2014; 128:291–303.
25. Kleinman CL, Gerges N, Papillon-Cavanagh S, et al. Fusion of TTYH1 with the C19MC microRNA cluster drives expression of a brain-specific DNMT3B isoform in the embryonal brain tumor ETMR. Nat Genet 2014; 46:39–44.
26. Schwalbe EC, Hayden JT, Rogers HA, et al. Histologically defined central nervous system primitive neuro-ectodermal tumours (CNS-PNETs) display heterogeneous DNA methylation profiles and show relationships to other paediatric brain tumour types. Acta Neuropathol 2013; 126:943–946.
27. Korshunov A, Capper D, Reuss D, et al. Histologically distinct neuroepithelial tumors with histone 3 G34 mutation are molecularly similar and comprise a single nosologic entity. Acta Neuropathol 2016; 131:137–146.
28. de Kock L, Sabbaghian N, Druker H, et al. Germ-line and somatic DICER1 mutations in pineoblastoma. Acta Neuropathol 2014; 128:583–595.
29. de Kock L, Sabbaghian N, Plourde F, et al. Pituitary blastoma: a pathognomonic feature of germ-line. Acta Neuropathol 2014; 128:1–12.

Chapter 9

The role of the autopsy in the diagnosis of sepsis and related fatal syndromes

Sebastian Lucas

INTRODUCTION

"The definition of sepsis, like pornography, was in the eyes of the beholder" (Robert Balk, [1]).

The major problems in the evaluation of clinical sepsis are the imprecision of case definitions and its subjectivity. Patients with sepsis – a severe infection associated with vital organ dysfunction – comprise a large proportion of the critically ill population. Although outcomes have improved, mortality is still >25%, and up to 50% when shock is present [2]. The bed costs of patients managed in UK critical care hospital settings are typically £1,500 per day; a pan-European study found the total cost of a sepsis case to be €25,000 [3] – amounting to a major proportion of national health systems' expenditure. In the UK, 65,000 people per annum survive severe sepsis, but there are long-term sequelae and a high medium-term mortality [2,4].

A significant proportion of deaths from sepsis will be autopsied, usually (in the UK) on request from a coroner or fiscal, or as a consented autopsy via interested clinicians in intensive care units (ICUs). Clinician–researchers' reviews of sepsis emphasise how little (macroscopically at least) there may be to see at autopsy in fatal cases [5] – though one aim of this overview is to depict how useful a critical examination of histology can be.

Sepsis is overdiagnosed clinically in life [6]. Thus, the roles of the autopsy are:

- To assess its presence and causation
- To consider alternative diagnoses that clinically simulate sepsis [7]
- To consider the impact of treatments for sepsis on outcome
- To contribute to research into the pathogenesis of sepsis

WHAT IS SEPSIS?

Case definitions of sepsis are needed to identify septic patients, to treat them optimally and to conduct clinical trials. Unfortunately, the current definitions have high sensitivity but low specificity: most patients in ICU will fulfil the current case definition whether or not they are septic [6].

Sebastian Lucas FRCP FRCPath Department of Histopathology, St Thomas' Hospital, London, UK

Sepsis is defined as the presence (probable or documented) of infection together with systemic manifestation of infection [8]. These manifestations are collectively termed SIRS – the systemic inflammatory response syndrome [1]. Severe sepsis is sepsis plus sepsis-induced organ dysfunction or tissue hypoperfusion. Septic shock is defined as sepsis-induced hypotension persisting despite adequate fluid resuscitation. **Table 9.1** expands on these clinical, physiological and laboratory data definitions (for precise values, see Dellinger [8]).

Feedback from autopsy information can usefully inform clinicians on the accuracy of their case definitions. Moreover, these definitions have been modified progressively since their introduction in 1991, constantly seeking better discrimination between those ill patients who are genuinely infected (septic) and those with SIRS due to non-infectious diseases.

EPIDEMIOLOGY OF SEPSIS

International estimates vary, due in part to different case definitions with approximately 300 cases per 100,000 population per annum [9]; thus in high-income countries, it is more common than myocardial infarction and stroke.

Sepsis develops either in the community, and patients arrive via emergency departments to hospital; or in hospital inpatients whose condition deteriorates. The estimate of community-origin sepsis is >70% of cases [10]; a small proportion of these die at home, en route to hospital or shortly after arrival, and most of these will become the subject of a medicolegal autopsy to determine the cause of death.

OUTCOMES OF SEPSIS

In addition to the high immediate mortality, which is related to the severity of the sepsis process and its cause, there are indirect and late complications whose significance is only now becoming appreciated. A study of elderly (median age: 77 years) survivors of severe sepsis found that 80% of them had died by 5 years after discharge [4]. Persistent critical illness (PCI) with significant morbidities is common after leaving the ICU (**Table 9.2**).

This suggests that 'recent survival from severe sepsis' can reasonably be inserted as a diagnosis into the part 2, or even part 1, of medical certificates of cause of death.

Table 9.1 The clinical and laboratory criteria of systemic inflammatory response syndrome (SIRS)	
The clinical type of variable	Abnormalities
General	Fever, hypothermia, tachycardia, tachypnoea, altered mental status, oedema, hyperglycaemia
Inflammatory	Leucocytosis, leukopaenia, normal wbc with many immature forms, elevated plasma c-reactive protein, elevated plasma calcitonin
Haemodynamic	Arterial hypotension
Organ dysfunction	Arterial hypoxaemia, acute lung injury, oliguria, raised creatinine, coagulopathy, ileus, thrombocytopaenia, hyperbilirubinaemia
Tissue perfusion	Hyperlactataemia, decreased capillary refill or skin mottling

Table 9.2 Persistent critical illnesses (PCI) after survival of sepsis [4,10]
Neurocognitive dysfunction
Functional chronic cardiorespiratory failure
Renal failure
Amputation
Neuropathies
Skeletal myopathy (leading to progressive sarcopaenia and frailty)
Immune dysfunction (leading to increased susceptibility to infection)

Table 9.3 Risk factors for sepsis	
General risk factors	**Specific risk factors**
Malignancy	Hyposplenism
Diabetes	Splenectomy
Alcohol abuse	Sickle cell disease
Autoimmune disorders	Congenital
Extremes of age	Liver cirrhosis
Obesity	HIV disease
	Immunosuppressive therapies
	Transplantation

RISK FACTORS FOR SEVERE SEPSIS

The extremes of age are well known to be major risk factors for sepsis, as exemplified by the U-shaped profile of incident cases of reported group A *Streptococcus* infection isolations with respect to age [11]. **Table 9.3** lists the more significant risk factors, general and specific.

The pathogeneses of these risk factors are mostly self-evident. Cancer and its treatments affect the immune system, innate and acquired, as do autoimmune disorders. Liver cirrhosis, of any cause, alters the haemodynamics in the liver, so that the Kupffer cells (which form 30% of all liver cells) are less well perfused and so do not remove toxic materials. Encouragingly, the high mortality of sepsis in cirrhotic patients has declined recently, due to better intensive care protocols [12]. Diabetes, HIV infection [13], immunosuppressive therapies (including transplantation) and the extremes of age all affect both immune systems' functions.

The biological contribution of morbid obesity to the risk of sepsis is controversial; what is not disputed are the increased practical difficulty in diagnosing infection in such patients (clinical features are obscured and delayed) and the operative problems involved in surgical interventions.

Hyposplenism, i.e. an absent, small or non-functioning fibrosed spleen, has a specific impact on resistance to encapsulated bacterial infection, of which the pneumococcus is the most important. Often due to sickle cell disease, it is major risk factor for bacterial infections in people with sickle cell disease in blood, lung, bone and meninges.

THE PATHOGENESIS OF SEPSIS AND SIRS

The more important infections that initiate sepsis in adults are listed in **Table 9.4**. Paediatric sepsis has a similar range of causative infections, and – like adults – culture investigations are negative in life in up to 40% of cases of sepsis and septic shock [2,14].

The pathogenesis of sepsis is complex and subject to intensive research [18]. The body's cells recognise infection through numerous receptors, e.g. toll-like receptors (TLR), and react to infection through the innate and the acquired immune systems' responses. These include production of cytokine messengers (e.g. interleukin-1 (IL-1)) and tumour necrosis factor-alpha (TNF-alpha); these go on to both activate and damage host cells and organs.

The critical end results in sepsis are [2]:

- Epithelial dysfunction
- Endothelial leakage
- Disrupted cellular metabolism
- Lymphocyte apoptosis

The current pathogenetic concepts emphasise sequential phases of overlapping networks of interactions, teleologically intended to benefit the host but potentially causing injury and death with balances and imbalances in the process [1,2,5,19].

- Phase 1: Local pro-inflammatory response (SIRS) at the site of infection to limit spread and injury
- Phase 2: Early compensatory anti-inflammatory response (CARS) to maintain immunological balance
- Phase 3: SIRS predominates over CARS, resulting in endothelial cell dysfunction, increased microvascular permeability and coagulopathy

Table 9.4 Common infections causing severe sepsis/SIRS syndromes with haemophagocytosis	
Infections – viral	Epstein–Barr virus (EBV), CMV, herpes simplex
	HIV
	Influenza – pandemic [16]
	Parvovirus B19
Infections – bacterial	*Streptococcus pyogenes* and *S. pneumoniae*
	Staphylococcus aureus (MSSA and MRSA)
	Rickettsia spp.
	Escherichia coli, *Klebsiella* spp. and other gram-negative bacilli
	Mycobacterium tuberculosis [17]
	Clostridium spp.
	Leptospira spp.
	Legionella spp.
Infections – fungal	*Histoplasma capsulatum*, *Candida*, *Aspergillus* spp.
Infections – parasitic	*Plasmodium falciparum*
	Leishmaniasis (*L. donovani*)
	Toxoplasma gondii in the immunosuppressed
Modified from Ramos-Casals et al [15].	

- Phase 4: CARS becomes excessive, resulting in immunodepression or immune paralysis (and pathologically, apoptosis of T cells); this can render the host susceptible to further nosocomial or secondary infections
- Phase 5: Multiple organ failure/dysfunction

In addition to cytokines from macrophages and T cells, the importance of adrenal steroids and the sympathetic nervous system in SIRS is underappreciated [5]. These concepts and the grades of sepsis (sepsis, severe sepsis and septic shock) are not matters that autopsy pathology can usually directly evaluate, and clinical and laboratory estimations are more important. The first two grades can be regarded as phasic failures of homeostasis, but septic shock is different in that – from experimental evidence as well as clinical studies – excessive TNFα is the major and necessary mediator [2,5]. The toxic shock syndrome (TSS) overlaps with septic shock clinically, but has another contributory pathogenesis: superantigens of *Streptococcus pyogenes* and *Staphylococcus aureus* activate circulating T cells to release cytokines that promote a self-accelerating release of pro-inflammatory cytokines [18].

Host–response genetics in sepsis

It is important to emphasise the variability of the host response to a 'standard' infection injury, whereby, for example, one person acquires group A *Streptococcus* skin infection that causes only a local self-limited reaction, while another develops septic shock and can be dead within a day. There may be a dose–response relation here, but more important is the status of the host's immune response genetic make-up. In autopsy practice, this emerges when trying to explain to relatives why a patient died despite a correct infection diagnosis, appropriate antibiotics and full ICU support.

Two examples of the genetic influences over host responses are:
- Polymorphisms related to CD14, a component of the innate immune system that brings about the recognition and binding of lipopolysaccharides (LPS, from gram-negative bacteria) to TLR [2].
- Variants in the FER gene associated with the reduced death rate in community-acquired pneumonia [20], raising the usual possibility that it might be a target for novel therapies.

Partial abnormalities of the perforin system that regulates T cells are also relevant to inherited risk of sepsis (see below). But we do not currently understand nor are able to identify most of an individual's host response factors, beyond the generic factors (**Table 9.3**).

CAUSES OF THE SIMULATORS OF SEVERE SEPSIS

The clinical features of severe sepsis are nonspecific. Most patients will be admitted to ICU, diagnostic samples taken and imaging performed; and then they are commenced on organ-support treatments and empirical antibiotics. Intensivists admit that they work primarily to restore patient physiology towards normal with perhaps less attention to identifying the underlying cause of the SIRS, i.e. they are scenario-driven rather than aetiology-driven. The proportion of patients diagnosed with severe sepsis who die but actually had a non-infectious pathogenesis is not known. No usual hospital discharge-coding system or national cause of death statistics could identify them; only single-centre or multicentre studies that combine detailed ICU clinical review with complete autopsy examination of all deaths could obtain the necessary data – and that is not going to happen anywhere.

Certain cancers, particularly T-cell and B-cell lymphomas, inaugurate a cytokine storm that triggers SIRS and haemophagocytosis (HPC), and hence multi-organ failure [21]. Frustratingly for clinicians, these tumours may be small and occult, and only diagnosed after death. Similarly many autoimmune diseases can, without obvious provocation, trigger fatal SIRS, particularly (in my experience) adult-onset Still's disease (AOSD) [22,23] and vasculitis [7]. Combining anecdotal autopsy observations and published studies from ICUs enables us to tabulate the range of these sepsis-simulating diseases. The haemophagocytic syndrome (HPCS) is the key defining feature.

CAUSES OF HPC

The HPCSs haemophagocytic lymphohistiocytosis (HLH) and macrophage activation syndrome (MAS)] have a wide range of causes, symptoms and outcomes, including fatality [15]. They all lead to a hyperinflammatory response and organ damage, i.e. the clinical features of severe sepsis, which is the leading cause of HPCS. Taxonomically, they are divided into primary (genetic) and secondary (reactive) categories. The former are mainly paediatric, and adults predominantly comprise the latter, driven most commonly by infections (see **Table 9.5**).

The inheritable contribution of perforin genes to HPCS and SIRS

Pathophysiologically, the common underlying mechanism in genetic forms of HPC is a defect in granule-mediated cytotoxicity. The inherited genetic defects include perforin gene on chromosome 9q21, the *MUNC13-4* gene on chromosome 17q25 or mutations in *syntaxin 11* gene on chromosome 6q24 [15,25]. The perforin and Fas systems maintain homeostasis of dendritic cells and restrict T-cell activation from antigen presentation. In HPCS, uncontrolled activation of antigen-presenting cells and T cells results in a cytokine storm with secretion of proinflammatory cytokines such as TNFα, IL-1 and IL-6. These activate macrophages and additionally cause the tissue damage that leads to multi-organ failure. The inherited forms present in childhood, but it is likely that partial loss of perforin and cytotoxic activity underlies many of the acquired, adult cases of severe HPCS; in other words, there is spectral genetic heterogeneity [25].

The categorisation of HPCS into genetic versus reactive has therapeutic implications: if it is primarily caused by a gene defect, treatment includes chemotherapy and bone marrow transplantation; if it is reactive, then treating the initiating condition plus intensive care is appropriate.

THE AUTOPSY PROCEDURE

There is considerable and repetitive literature comparing pre- and postmortem autopsy findings in patients who die in ICU with sepsis, perioperative complications and trauma [26]. As well as those noting the still-high proportion of clinically undiagnosed or treated-but-persistent infections [27], there are also focussed studies that, for example, compare the clinical diagnosis with autopsy diagnosis of ventilator-associated pneumonia (VAP) [28]. All studies emphasise the quality control aspect of post-ICU and sepsis autopsy examination with up to one third of patients having significant infections as well as other problems that were underappreciated in life [29]. Among the infections, occult but fatal

Table 9.5 The noninfective reactive triggers of HPC in adults	
Neoplasms – haematological	T-cell lymphoma
	B-cell lymphoma
	Hodgkin disease
	Leukaemias
	Multicentric Castleman disease (MCCD) [24]
	Some carcinomas
Autoimmune diseases	Systemic lupus erythematosus (SLE)
	Adult-onset Still's disease (AOSD)
	Rheumatoid arthritis
	Systemic vasculitis of medium and small vessels
Transplantation	Solid organ
	Haematological
Other	Sickle cell disease (splenic hyperhaemolysis syndrome)
	Drug treatments
	Surgery, e.g. bypass vascular surgery
	Vaccination
	Haemodialysis
	Pancreatitis
	Burns
	Major trauma
	Heat stroke
	Thyroid storm
	Thrombotic thrombocytopaenic purpura (TTP)
Unknown	'Idiopathic'
Adapted from Ramos-Casals et al [15].	

fungal infections [30], such as aspergillosis, herpes simplex and mycobacterial disease are recurrent items.

Many of the infections that cause death from systemic sepsis are evident from standard careful examination of the major organ systems, such as meningitis, pneumonia, peritonitis, urosepsis, genital tract sepsis [31] and biliary sepsis [27]. And the predisposing factors may also be evident, such as perforation of hollow viscus, gall stones, tumours, sinusitis, etc.

There is also gross pathology that relates to sepsis arising not in a visible focus of infection but indirectly from blood infection alone, such as adrenal haemorrhage in meningococcaemia and other bacteraemias (the Waterhouse–Friedrichsen syndrome, although most septic adrenal haemorrhages are more microscopic than gross). The source of entry of virulent bacteria into the body may be evident, for example, from a skin rash, not always very obvious, which on histology is cellulitis or early necrotising fasciitis containing vast numbers of gram-positive cocci as in group A streptococcal infection.

One 'pathology' often touted as diagnostic of sepsis is the 'diffluent spleen.' My own observations of autopsy spleens that, when cut, pour out their contents as a red soup, are found more often in patients that had not been in severe sepsis than had; and the most important cause of spleen diffluence is postmortem autolysis.

However, in many cases of overwhelming SIRS multi-organ failure, there is little to see grossly beyond soft, red and congested organs (**Figure 9.1**)

INVESTIGATIONS FOR SEPSIS AT AUTOPSY

Many microbiological tests will usually have been undertaken in life, so it is essential to obtain a full record of these, alongside the haematology data (for coagulation abnormalities) and relevant biochemistry. Some patients will have had biopsies and organ resections, which must be reviewed (at least on paper).

A lot of useful microbiology can be performed on material at autopsy. **Table 9.6** lists the most useful samples. Blood culture sampling should be done before the body is opened, and blood taken from neck veins or heart; any blood samples from below the umbilicus are liable to be contaminated by faeces. Cerebrospinal fluid can be taken from either the L4-5 space or the cisterna magna (below the occipital process on the neck). Sampling internal organs without contamination is inevitably difficult; use new clean instruments and consult with microbiologists if the culture results are confusing.

INTERPRETATION OF THE AUTOPSY HISTOPATHOLOGY

By now, it is evident that for a comprehensive appreciation of sepsis (and related scenarios) at autopsy, a full set of tissues must be examined histologically in addition to appropriate cultures of blood and/or infective foci in organs [33].

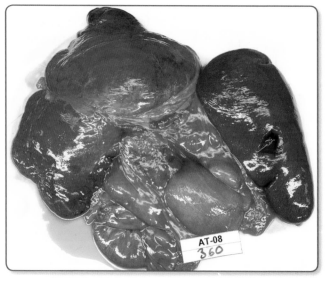

Figure 9.1 Toxic shock syndrome caused by group A streptococcal blood infection, resulting in enlarged, soggy, red abdominal organs.

Table 9.6 Microbiological and immunological sampling for infection at autopsy		
Material	Tests	Practical notes
Blood for culture	Aerobic and anaerobic bacteria, fungi, mycobacteria	
Blood for molecular PCR diagnostics	Meningococcus Pneumococcus	
Blood/serum for serology	HIV	Essential if not known but suspected
Blood/serum for cytokine analysis	Endotoxin	Still being validated [32]
Urine	Pneumococcal antigen Legionella antigen	
Focal organ tissue: sepsis culture and molecular diagnostics	Bacteria, fungi, mycobacteria	Molecular diagnostics are the future optimum but variably available. Increasingly, molecular diagnostics can be performed on formalin-fixed paraffin-embedded (FFPE) material
Faeces	Bacteria	
Cerebrospinal fluid (CSF)	Bacteria, mycobacteria, fungi – cytopreparations and culture	
Any tissue	Cytology dab preparations	Giemsa stain is better than Papanicolau, plus standard infection stains

Specific infection identification

The identification of many specific infections can be achieved through histopathology alone (though culture, and molecular technologies are always appropriate for confirmation): pneumococci (**Figure 9.2**), many mycobacteria, *Listeria*, *Leishmania donovani* (an under-recognised cause of HPCS and sometimes death, **Figure 9.3**) are examples. Fungal infections can be difficult; many are recognised on histology, but there are many similar morphologies and the treatment increasingly depends on correct generic identification. Molecular diagnostics is now becoming as or more important than culture in speed and accuracy [30].

In the lung, the low sensitivity of pathologists in diagnosing bronchopneumonia by gross examination compared with gold standard histopathology is well known [34]. Neutropaenic sepsis involving the lung manifests few or no neutrophil polymorphs but abundant bacteria or fungi (usually *Aspergillus* spp. causing necrosis by obstructing blood vessels). The accurate diagnosis of acute lung injury (diffuse alveolar damage) is impossible without histopathology.

General pathology features

Other critical observations (relating to **Table 9.3**) include the presence of diabetes (kidney microvascular damage), alcoholic and end-stage liver disease (cirrhosis), sickle cell disease (sickled red cells in blood vessels) and HIV infection (often diagnosable on histology if not previously treated [35]).

Thrombotic microangiopathies (TMA) are broadly divided into disseminated intravascular coagulation (DIC) and thrombotic thrombocytopaenia purpura (TTP)

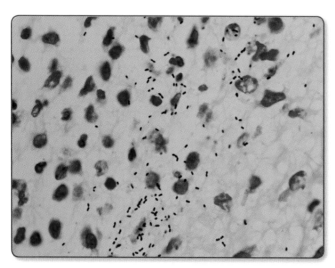

Figure 9.2 Pneumococcal meningitis (Streptococcus pneumoniae). The gram-positive diplococci are diagnostic (Gram, oil immersion).

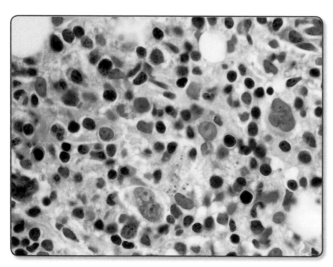

Figure 9.3 Visceral leishmaniasis causing fatal haemophagocytosis. The parasites are seen as small blue dots in the central macrophages (H&E, oil immersion).

syndromes. DIC is a feature of many cases of severe sepsis with coagulopathy, best seen in the glomerular and lung alveolar capillaries. TTP, on the other hand, is not a feature of sepsis, although it can mimic it clinically, and the thrombi are seen in kidney, heart, lung and brain vessels. If there is doubt as to the type of TMA present, immunostains resolve the problem: DIC is strongly fibrin positive with some platelets present (using anti-CD61); TTP is almost entirely composed of platelets with minimal fibrin.

SIRS histopathology

Many of the useful histopathological features seen in SIRS due to severe sepsis and its simulator diseases are indicated in **Table 9.7**. In my experience, the most useful are:

- Haemophagocytosis (**Figures 9.4** and **9.5**)
- Upregulated intercellular adhesion molecule-1 (ICAM-1) expression in lung endothelial cells [36] (**Figure 9.6**)
- Lymphopaenia in spleen and lymph nodes [37] (**Figure 9.7**)

Table 9.7 The generic histopathological features (i.e. not direct observation of an infection) that support a diagnosis of SIRS		
Tissue	Histopathology	Practical notes
Lung	DIC	
	Acute lung injury	
	ICAM-1 expression in endothelial cells (with CD54 immunostain)	Reflects TNFα and inflammatory cytokine effect; normal lung endothelia are negative
Liver	Cholestasis	
	Cholangiolitis	
	Kupffer cell hyperplasia and haemophagocytosis	Best seen with CD68 IHC for macrophages
	Unusually advanced autolysis	A consequence of TNFα circulating at death
Kidney	DIC	Common in meningococcaemia; differential diagnosis = TTP
Spleen	White pulp atrophy	Apoptosis often evident
	Fibrinoid necrosis around small follicles	
	Red pulp haemophagocytosis	Best seen with CD68 IHC
Bone marrow	Haemophagocytosis	Best seen with CD68 IHC. In persons surviving sepsis for weeks before death, the haemopoietic marrow may atrophy, although the HPC remains
Lymph nodes	Lymphopaenia and increased apoptosis of lymphocytes	
Heart	Interstitial oedema and prominence of mononuclear cells	To be distinguished from true myocarditis by Dallas criteria
	ICAM-1 expression in endothelial cells (CD54)	

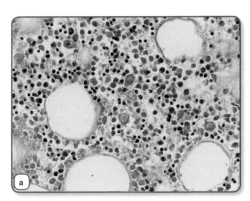
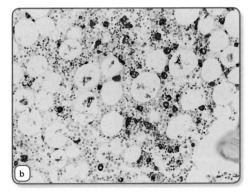

Figure 9.4 Haemophagocytosis in marrow in streptococcal sepsis. (a) Bone marrow macrophages are increased in number, enlarged and contain multiple nuclei or cell fragments; despite autolysis, at least six such macrophages are visible (H&E). (b) CD68 (PGM-1) immunostain highlights the enlarged phagocytosing macrophages.

Treatment complications

Beyond organ support, fluid balance and antibiotics, research into better treatment of sepsis has sought more precise molecular targets in sepsis pathogenesis [2]. The therapeutic alternatives for infective versus non-infective HPCSs have already been

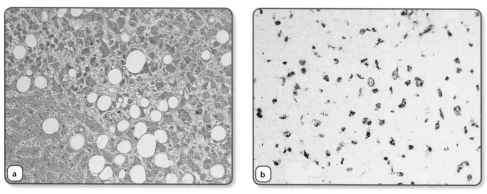

Figure 9.5 Haemophagocytosis in liver in fatal leptospirosis. (a) The liver appears autolysed and featureless apart from steatosis and some cholestasis (H&E). (b) Same case with CD68 immunostain: the abundant enlarged phagocytosing Kupffer cells are highlighted.

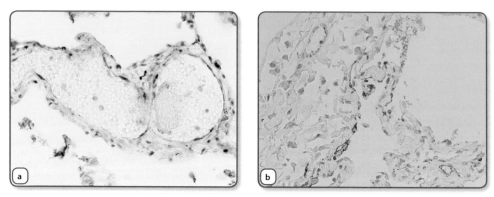

Figure 9.6 (a,b) Upregulation of intercellular adhesion molecule-1 (ICAM-1) in the cytoplasm of lung endothelial cells. Two different cases are illustrated. There is always epithelial cell staining, which is to be ignored (CD54 immunostain).

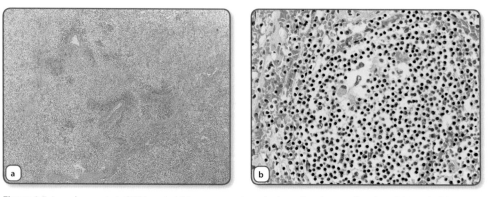

Figure 9.7 Lymphopaenia in SIRS/sepsis. (a) Low power view of spleen showing small periarterial lymphoid (white) pulp (H&E). (b) Apoptosis process with lymphocyte fragments in the imploding lymphoid follicle (H&E, oil immersion).

described. The number of agents being considered is huge: drugs targeting epithelial barriers and endothelial function, drugs aimed at interrupting specific immune activation sites and at improving sepsis-related immunosuppression, and drugs and vaccines aimed more generally at the prevention of sepsis level – many are at preclinical and trial status. Many of these agents have potential pathological side effects, and autopsy pathology can contribute to their recognition. One example, where a sepsis treatment had to be dropped, is activated protein C (aPC): the risk of major organ haemorrhage (in brain and lung) due to the drug's action outweighed any benefit it produced in survival [38]. However, there is no 'magic bullet' drug that can modify all types of severe sepsis.

CONCLUSION

The autopsy has a major role in evaluating deaths in clinical sepsis, by identifying causative agents [10], determining whether a non-infective disease caused an apparent 'sepsis' death and looking for complications of intensive care, i.e. pathology as quality control. But the procedure must be done rigorously with appropriate investigations and with a broad knowledge of modern medicine and its practice. In particular, by carefully depicting and categorising these complex deaths, pathologists contribute to our evolving knowledge of the inheritable factors that determine the risk of severe sepsis.

One specific feedback message to our clinical colleagues, faced with apparent severe sepsis but of unknown aetiology, is to urge them to obtain critical tissue for diagnosis: a bone marrow trephine biopsy (not aspirate) and the biggest lymph node accessible [7].

Key points for clinical practice

- The diagnosis in most sepsis-related autopsies will be made on a combination of clinical, imaging, laboratory and pathological data and integration.
- Obtain the results of all premortem laboratory tests, if done.
- Take microbiology samples from blood and any obvious infected sites.
- Take a full set of histopathology, including bone marrow from vertebrae.
- Apply immunohistochemical stains to highlight the effects of cytokines on organs.
- Think whether the death was due to infection or a simulator of clinical sepsis.

REFERENCES

1. Balk RA. Systemic inflammatory response syndrome (SIRS). Where did it come from and is it still relevant today? Virulence 2014; 5:20–26.
2. Cohen J, Vincent JL, Adhikari NKJ, et al. Sepsis: a road-map for future research. Lancet Infect Dis 2015; 15:581–614.
3. Vincent JL, Sakr Y, Sprung CL, et al. Sepsis in European intensive care units: results of the SOAP study. Crit Care Med 2006; 34:344–353.
4. Iwashnya TJ, Ely EW, Smith DM, et al. Long-term cognitive impairment and functional disability among survivors of severe sepsis. JAMA 2010; 304:1787–1794.
5. Deutschmann CS, Tracey KJ. Sepsis: current dogma and new perspectives. Immunity 2014; 40:463–475.
6. Vincent JL, Opal SM, Marshall JC, et al. Sepsis definitions: time for a change. Lancet 2013; 381:774–775.
7. Lucas SB. Sepsis definitions. Lancet 2013; 381:2249.

8.   Dellinger RP, Levy MM, Rhodes A, et al. Surviving sepsis campaign: International Guidelines for Management of Severe Sepsis and Septic Shock: 2012. Crit Care Med 2013; 41:580–637.

9.   Hall MJ, Williams SN, DeFrances CJ, et al. Inpatient care for septicemia or sepsis: a challenge for patients and hospitals. NCHS Data Brief, Number 62. USA: Centers for Disease Control and Prevention, 2011.

10. National Confidential Enquiry into Patient Outcome and Death (NCEPOD). Review of the care received by patients with sepsis. London: NCEPOD, 2015.

11. O'Loughlin RE, Roberson A, Cieslak PR et al. The epidemiology of invasive Group A Streptococcal infection and potential vaccine implications: United States, 2000-2004. Clin Infect Dis 2007; 45:853-862.

12. Galbois A, Aegerter P, Martel-Samb P, et al. Improved prognosis of septic shock in patients with cirrhosis: a multicentre study. Crit Care Med 2014; 42:1666–1675.

13. Huson MAM, Grobusch MP, van der Pall T. The effect of HIV infection on host response to bacterial sepsis. Lancet Infect Dis 2015; 15:109–121.

14. Schlapbach LJ, Straney L, Alexander J, et al. Mortality related to invasive infections, sepsis, and septic shock in critically ill children in Australia and New Zealand, 2002-13: a multicentre retrospective cohort study. Lancet Infect Dis 2015; 15:46–54.

15. Ramos-Casals M, Brito-Zeron P, Lopez-Guillermo A, et al. Adult haemophagocytic syndrome. Lancet 2014; 383:1503–1516.

16. Lucas SB. Predictive clinicopathological features derived from systematic autopsy examination of patients who died with A/H1N1 influenza infection in the UK 2009-10. Health Technol Assess 2010; 14:83–114.

17. Brastianos PK, Swanson JW, Torbenson M, et al. Tuberculosis-associated haemophagocytic syndrome. Lancet Infect Dis 2006; 6:447–454.

18. Munford RS, Suffredini AF. Sepsis, severe sepsis and septic shock. In: Mandell GL, Bennett JE, Dolin R (eds), Mandell, Douglas, and Bennett's principles and practice of infectious diseases, 7th edn. Philadelphia, PA: Churchill Livingstone, 2010:987–1010.

19. Bone RC, Grodzin CJ, Balk RA. Sepsis: a new hypothesis for pathogenesis of the disease process. Chest 1997; 112:235–248.

20. Rautanen A, Mills TC, Gordon AC, et al. Genome-wide association study of survival from sepsis due to pneumonia: an observational cohort study. Lancet Resp Med 2015; 3:53–60.

21. Alomari A, Hui P, Xu M. Composite peripheral T-cell lymphoma, NOS, and B-cell small lymphocytic lymphoma presenting with hemophagocytic lymphohistiocytosis. Int Surg Pathol 2013; 21:303–308.

22. Kumakura S, Ishikura H, Kondo M, et al. Autoimmune-associated haemophagocytic syndrome. Mod Rheumatol 2004; 14:205–215.

23. Atteritano M, David A, Bagnato G, et al. Haemophagocytic syndrome in rheumatic patients. A systematic review. Eur Rev Med Pharmmacol Sci 2012; 16:1414–1424.

24. Mylona EE, Baraboutis IG, Lekakis LJ, et al. Multicentric Castleman's disease in HIV infection: a systematic review of the literature. AIDS Rev 2008; 10:25–35.

25. Castillo L, Carcillo J. Secondary haemophagocytic lymphohistiocytosis and severe sepsis/systemic inflammatory response syndrome/multiorgan dysfunction syndrome/macrophage activation syndrome share common intermediate phenotypes on a spectrum of inflammation. Pediatr Crit Care Med 2009; 10:387–392.

26. Blosser SA, Zimmerman HE, Stauffer JL. Do autopsies of critically ill patients reveal important findings that were clinically undetected? Crit Care Med 1998; 26:1332–1336.

27. Torgersen C, Moser P, Luckner G, et al. Macroscopic post-mortem findings in 235 surgical intensive care patients with sepsis. Crit Care Trauma 2009; 108:1841–1847.

28. Fabregas N, Ewig S, Torres A, et al. Clinical diagnosis of ventilator associated pneumonia revisited: comparative validation using immediate post-mortem lung biopsies. Thorax 1999; 54:867–873.

29. De Vlieger GYA, Mahieu EMJ, Meersseman W. Clinical review: what is the role for autopsy in the ICU? Crit Care 2010; 14:221.

30. Schelenz S, Barnes RA, Barton RC, et al. British Society for Medical Mycology best practice recommendations for the diagnosis of serious fungal diseases. Lancet Infect Dis 2015; 15:461–474.

31. Lucas SB. The maternal death autopsy. In: Pignatelli M, Gallagher P (eds), Recent advances in histopathology, vol. 23. London: JP Medical Publishers, 2014:17–29.

32. Zhu BL, Ishikawa T, Michiue T, et al. Postmortem serum endotoxin level in relation to causes of death. Leg Med (Tokyo) 2005; 7:103–109.

33. Lucas SB. The autopsy pathology of sepsis-related death. In: Fernandez R (ed.), Severe sepsis and septic shock – understanding a serious killer. Rijeka: InTech, 2012.

34. Hunt CR, Benbow EW, Knox WF, et al. Can histopathologists diagnose bronchopneumonia? J Clin Pathol 1995; 48:120–123.
35. Mahadeva U, van der Walt JD, Moonim MT, et al. P24 immunohistochemistry on lymphoid tissue: the histopathologist's role in HIV diagnosis. Histopathology 2010; 56:542–547.
36. Tsokos M. Postmortem diagnosis of sepsis. Forensic Sci Int 2007; 165:155–164.
37. Hotchkiss RS, Earl IE. The pathophysiology and treatment of sepsis. N Eng J Med 2003; 348:138–150.
38. Martí-Carvajal AJ, Solà I, Lathyris D, Cardona AF. Human recombinant activated protein C for severe sepsis. Cochrane Database Syst Rev 2012; 3:CD004388.